Clinicians' Guides to Radionuclide Hybrid Imaging

PET/CT

Series Editors

Jamshed B. Bomanji
London, UK

Gopinath Gnanasegaran
London, UK

Stefano Fanti
Bologna, Italy

Homer A. Macapinlac
Houston, Texas, USA

More information about this series at http://www.springernature.com/series/13803

Sobhan Vinjamuri
Editor

PET/CT in Thyroid Cancer

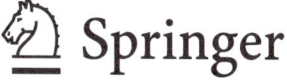
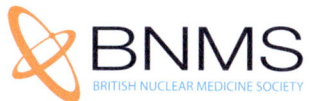

Editor
Sobhan Vinjamuri
Department of Nuclear Medicine
Royal Liverpool and Broadgreen University
Hospitals NHS Trust
Liverpool
UK

ISSN 2367-2439   ISSN 2367-2447 (electronic)
Clinicians' Guides to Radionuclide Hybrid Imaging - PET/CT
ISBN 978-3-319-71845-3   ISBN 978-3-319-71846-0 (eBook)
https://doi.org/10.1007/978-3-319-71846-0

Library of Congress Control Number: 2018930909

© Springer International Publishing AG, part of Springer Nature 2018
This work is subject to copyright. All rights are reserved by the Publisher, whether the whole or part of the material is concerned, specifically the rights of translation, reprinting, reuse of illustrations, recitation, broadcasting, reproduction on microfilms or in any other physical way, and transmission or information storage and retrieval, electronic adaptation, computer software, or by similar or dissimilar methodology now known or hereafter developed.
The use of general descriptive names, registered names, trademarks, service marks, etc. in this publication does not imply, even in the absence of a specific statement, that such names are exempt from the relevant protective laws and regulations and therefore free for general use.
The publisher, the authors and the editors are safe to assume that the advice and information in this book are believed to be true and accurate at the date of publication. Neither the publisher nor the authors or the editors give a warranty, express or implied, with respect to the material contained herein or for any errors or omissions that may have been made. The publisher remains neutral with regard to jurisdictional claims in published maps and institutional affiliations.

Printed on acid-free paper

This Springer imprint is published by the registered company Springer International Publishing AG part of Springer Nature
The registered company address is: Gewerbestrasse 11, 6330 Cham, Switzerland

PET/CT series is dedicated to Prof Ignac Fogelman, Dr Muriel Buxton-Thomas and Prof Ajit K Padhy

Foreword

Clear and concise clinical indications for PET/CT in the management of oncology patient are presented in this series of 15 separate booklets.

Early and accurate diagnosis, better staging, tailored management and specific treatment of cancer in patients have been achieved with the advent of this multimodality imaging technology. Clear information on treatment responses can be collected using PET/CT, as well as prognostic information, which can serve as a guide for additional therapeutic options.

PET/CT was fortunately able to derive a great benefit from radionuclide-labelled probes, which deliver often excellent target and non-target signals. Whilst labelled glucose remains the cornerstone for the clinical benefit achieved, a number of recent probes are definitely adding benefit. PET/CT is hence an evolving technology with extensive applications and indications. Significant advances in the instrumentation and data processing available have also contributed to this technology, which delivers a wealth of high-throughput data, is well tolerated by patients and indeed is accepted by patients and the public. As an example, the role of PET/CT in the evaluation of cardiac disease is also covered, with emphasis on labelled rubidium and labelled glucose studies.

The novel probes of labelled choline; labelled peptides, such as DOTATATE; and, most recently, labelled PSMA (prostate-specific membrane antigen) have gained rapid clinical utility and acceptance as significant PET/CT tools for the management of patients with neuroendocrine diseases and prostate cancer, notwithstanding all the advances achieved with other imaging modalities, such as MRI. Hence, a chapter reviewing novel PET tracers forms part of this series.

The oncological community has recognised the value of PET/CT and has delivered advanced diagnostic criteria for some of the most important indications for PET/CT. This includes the recent Deauville criteria for the classification of PET/CT patients with lymphoma, and similar criteria are expected to be developed for other malignancies, such as head and neck cancer, melanoma and pelvic malignancies. Finally, a separate section covers the role of PET/CT in radiotherapy planning, discussing the indications for planning biological tumour volumes in relevant cancers.

These booklets offer simple, rapid and concise guidelines on the utility of PET/CT in a range of oncological indications. They also deliver a rapid aide memoire on the merits and appropriate indications for PET/CT in oncology.

London, UK   Peter J. Ell, FMedSci, DR HC, AΩA

Preface

Hybrid imaging with PET/CT and SPECT/CT combines the best in function and structure to provide accurate localisation, characterisation and diagnosis. There is extensive literature and evidence to support PET/CT, which has made a significant impact in oncological imaging and management of patients with cancer. The evidence in favour of SPECT/CT especially in orthopaedic indications is evolving and increasing.

The *Clinicians' Guides to Radionuclide Hybrid Imaging* (PET/CT and SPECT/CT) pocketbook series is specifically aimed for referring clinicians, nuclear medicine/radiology doctors, radiographers/technologists and nurses who are routinely working in nuclear medicine and participate in multidisciplinary meetings. This series is a joint work of many friends and professionals from different nations who share a common dream and vision towards promoting and supporting nuclear medicine as a useful and important imaging speciality.

We want to thank all those people who have contributed to this work as advisors, authors and reviewers, without whom this book would not have been possible, and our members from the BNMS (British Nuclear Medicine Society, UK) for their encouragement and support. We are also extremely grateful to Dr. Brian Nielly, Charlotte Weston, the BNMS Education Committee and the BNMS council members for their enthusiasm and trust.

Finally, we wish to extend particular gratitude to the industry for their continuous supports towards education and training.

London, UK   Gopinath Gnanasegaran
                                                        Jamshed Bomanji

Acknowledgements

The series co-ordinators and editors would like to express sincere gratitude to the members of the British Nuclear Medicine Society, patients, teachers, colleagues, students, the industry and the BNMS Education Committee Members for their continued support and inspiration.

Andy Bradley
Brent Drake
Francis Sundram
James Ballinger
Parthiban Arumugam
Rizwan Syed
Sai Han
Vineet Prakash

Contents

1. **Thyroid Cancer** 1
   Susannah L. Shore

2. **Thyroid Cancer Pathology** 9
   Susannah L. Shore

3. **Management of Thyroid Cancer** 15
   M.P. Rowland, A.J. Waghorn, and S. Vinjamuri

4. **Radiological Imaging in Thyroid Cancer** 25
   Rashika Fernando

5. **Radionuclide Imaging in Thyroid Cancer** 35
   Emmanouil Panagiotidis

6. **^{18}F-FDG PET/CT Normal Variants, Artefacts and Pitfalls in Thyroid Cancer** 45
   Arun Sasikumar, Alexis Corrigan, Muhammad Umar Khan, and Gopinath Gnanasegaran

7. **Metabolic PET/CT Imaging in Thyroid Cancer** 61
   Ioan Prata

8. **Benign and Malignant Thyroid Diseases on ^{18}F FDG PET/CT: Pictorial Atlas** 67
   Haseeb Ahmed and Hosahalli Mohan

Index 83

Contributors

Haseeb Ahmed Department of Nuclear Medicine, Guy's & St Thomas' NHS Foundation Trust, London, UK

Alexis Corrigan Consultant in Radionuclide Radiology, Maidstone Hospital, Maidstone, UK

Rashika Fernando Royal Liverpool and Broadgreen University Hospitals NHS Trust, London, UK

Gopinath Gnanasegaran Department of Nuclear Medicine, Royal Free London NHS Foundation Trust, London, UK

Muhammad Umar Khan Al-Jahra Hospital, Al-Jahra, Kuwait

Hosahalli Mohan Department of Nuclear Medicine, Guy's & St Thomas' NHS Foundation Trust, London, UK

Emmanouil Panagiotidis Department of Nuclear Medicine, Royal Liverpool University Hospital, Liverpool, UK

Ioan Prata Bradford Teaching Hospitals NHS Foundation Trust, Bradford, United Kingdom

M.P. Rowland Department of Surgery, Royal Liverpool University Hospital, Liverpool, UK

Arun Sasikumar Consultant and Head of the Department, Department of Nuclear Medicine, St Gregorios International Cancer Care Centre, Parumala, Kerala, India

Susannah L. Shore Royal Liverpool and Broadgreen University Hospitals NHS Trust, Liverpool, UK

Sobhan Vinjamuri Department of Nuclear Medicine, Royal Liverpool and Broadgreen University Hospitals NHS Trust, Liverpool, UK

A.J. Waghorn Department of Surgery, Royal Liverpool University Hospital, Liverpool, UK

Thyroid Cancer

Susannah L. Shore

Contents

1.1 Clinical Presentation 2
1.2 Investigation and Classification of Thyroid Nodules 3
1.3 Staging and Prognosis of Differentiated Thyroid Cancer (DTC) 4
1.4 Summary 7
References 7

Thyroid cancer is the most common endocrine cancer yet only the 20th most common cancer in the UK and represents less than 1% of all new malignancies. There are three main types: papillary, follicular and medullary thyroid cancer. However, within these groups are many histological subtypes, which will be discussed in more detail in Chap. 2. Rarely thyroid cancer can be anaplastic cancers which have a very poor prognosis compared with all other types of thyroid cancer. Lymphoma of the thyroid can also occur; however, the treatment is with chemotherapy and will not be discussed further. The European incidence of thyroid cancer has increased in the last decade by 65% in women and 69% in men [1]. While this may be partially explained by increased diagnosis of micropapillary thyroid cancers due to increasing neck ultrasounds [2–4], there is data to suggest that all stages of thyroid cancer have increased [2] therefore implying that the actual incidence of thyroid cancer is increasing. 2011 cancer statistics reveal the age-standardised incidence of thyroid cancer has risen to 5.6 per 100,000 in women and 2.2 per 100,000 in men in the UK [1].

The prognosis of papillary and follicular thyroid cancer remains generally excellent and is currently stratified into low-, moderate- and high-risk cancers. The risk factors for thyroid cancer are female patients (2–3× male patients), radiation

---

S.L. Shore
Royal Liverpool and Broadgreen University Hospitals NHS Trust, Liverpool, UK
e-mail: Susannah.shore@rlbuht.nhs.uk

© Springer International Publishing AG, part of Springer Nature 2018
S. Vinjamuri (ed.), *PET/CT in Thyroid Cancer*, Clinicians' Guides to Radionuclide Hybrid Imaging, https://doi.org/10.1007/978-3-319-71846-0_1

Table 1.1 Thyroid cancer syndromes [5, 6]

Thyroid cancer syndrome	Gene mutation	Type of thyroid cancer	Associated features	Action
Multiple endocrine neoplasia (MEN) 2a	RET oncogene (codon 634 in >70%)	Medullary thyroid cancer	Phaeochromocytoma (40–60%) Hyperparathyroidism (10–30%)	Thyroidectomy before 5 years depending on codon
MEN 2b	RET oncogene (918,883 codon 98%)	Medullary thyroid cancer	Phaeochromocytomas (40–60%) Neuromas of the tongue Ganglioneuromas of intestines Marfanoid features	Thyroidectomy in the first year of life
Familial medullary thyroid cancer	RET oncogene (>95%)	Medullary thyroid cancer		
Familial papillary thyroid cancer (FPTC)	Gene unknown (inheritance of two and three is autosomal dominance)	Papillary thyroid cancer	1. FPTC + renal papillary tumour 2. FPTC +/− oxyphilia 3. FPTC in multinodular goitre	Three or more first-degree relatives

Table 1.2 Genetic syndromes associated with an increased risk of non-medullary thyroid cancer [5]

Familial syndrome	Gene mutation	Incidence of thyroid cancer (%)	Type of thyroid cancer
Cowden's syndrome	PTEN tumour suppressor gene	>10–35	Usually follicular, occasionally papillary
Familial adenomatous polyposis (FAP)	APC tumour suppressor gene	2–12	Papillary
Carney's complex	PRKAR1-x	4 and 60	Follicular and papillary, respectively
Werner's syndrome	WRN gene	18	Follicular anaplastic cancer

exposure especially in childhood (head and neck radiotherapy, mantle radiotherapy or nuclear fallout), family history of thyroid cancer (Table 1.1), endemic goitre, thyroid nodules and associated genetic syndromes [5] (Table 1.2).

1.1 Clinical Presentation

Thyroid cancer most commonly presents with a lump in the neck, usually anteriorly in the thyroid, but can, less commonly, present with a lateral neck lymph node. While a palpable thyroid nodule is a common finding (3–7%) [7] and requires investigation, only a small proportion (<5%) of these will turn out to be thyroid cancer. On ultrasound, nodules may be present in 30–70% of patients depending on age [8]. Concerning clinical features associated with a thyroid nodule or goitre include:

A male patient
Change in voice (hoarse or weak breathy voice) consistent with a recurrent laryngeal nerve (RLN) palsy
Compression symptoms (dyspnoea)
Stridor (from RLN palsy due to tumour invasion or large compressive goitre/tumour)
A rapidly enlarging thyroid nodule or a long-standing goitre increasing in size (in the presence of long-standing hypothyroidism, may indicate lymphoma)
A hard nodule or one fixed to the surrounding structures
The presence of cervical lymphadenopathy

Thyroid cancer can also present with symptoms from metastatic lesions especially vascular follicular bone lesions, which may present with cord compression or bone pain, multiple lung lesions found incidentally or liver lesions found incidentally or secondary to deranged liver function tests. More unusually skin lesions can be seen such as a hypervascular pulsatile swelling over the sternum, with a bruit or sometimes a palpable thrill.

1.2　Investigation and Classification of Thyroid Nodules

The investigation of thyroid cancer depends on the initial site of presentation. This is best performed within a specialist thyroid clinic. After a history and examination to identify any of the suspicious features discussed above, an ultrasound +/− fine needle aspiration cytology (FNAC) biopsy should be performed. Previously, a dominant nodule would undergo a FNAC biopsy based on size criteria. The Kim criteria for ultrasound assessment [9] are considered to have higher sensitivity and the American Association of Clinical Endocrinologists guidelines [10] have higher specificity. However, the most recent British Thyroid Association (BTA) Thyroid Cancer Guidelines 2014 [6] suggest a more formalised approach to the assessment of nodules with nodules being graded U1–U5 on ultrasound. U1 is normal and U5 malignant. Size alone has been shown to not correlate well with malignancy on ultrasound [11], but other ultrasound features including a non-smooth margin, an eccentric location of the solid portion, hypoechogenicity of the solid portion or the presence of micro-calcification within the solid portion of the nodule do correlate well with malignancy and have been incorporated into a visual U1–U5 guidance for radiologists as per the BTA guidance [6]. The overall shape is an important predictor of malignancy particularly if the nodule is taller than it is wide and for cystic/solid nodules if the shape is irregular in nature [12]. Indeterminate (U3) nodules and those suspicious of malignancy (U4–U5) require an FNAC biopsy. There has also been an increase in thyroid nodules diagnosed incidentally on CT and

^{18}fluoro-deoxy-glucose positron emission tomography (FDG PET) scan. CT is a poor modality for assessing thyroid nodules, but increased uptake on an FDG PET confers a >30% malignancy risk [13] and requires ultrasound assessment and FNAC.

The Royal College of Pathologists has produced guidance for the assessment of thyroid cytology [14]. The guidance categorises thyroid cytology as Thy1–Thy5 with Thy1 being inadequate, Thy2 benign, Thy3 indeterminate and divided into two categories (Thy3A and Thy3F), Thy4 suspicious of malignancy and Thy5 malignant. The risk of malignancy increases with each category from Thy2 up to Thy5. Thy1 is inadequate for assessment and requires a repeat FNAC. A patient with a thyroid nodule with a Thy2 cytology biopsy and a U2 benign ultrasound can be reassured and discharged. However, if the clinical suspicion or ultrasound appearances do not match a benign FNAC, then a repeat FNAC should be performed. MDT discussion is recommended for Thy4 and Thy5 nodules, but Thy3A and Thy3F categories will also benefit from an MDT discussion [6]. Thy3F and Thy4 nodules can undergo repeat cytology in an attempt to upgrade the diagnosis or undergo diagnostic surgery. A patient with a Thy5 cytology should undergo definitive surgery [6].

1.3 Staging and Prognosis of Differentiated Thyroid Cancer (DTC)

The prognosis of papillary and follicular thyroid cancer is generally very good. Even though there is a 5–20% risk of recurrence and 10–15% risk of distant metastases, only 9% of patients with DTC will die of their disease. Certain factors are known to be important in assessing prognosis and the risk of recurrence or death. These prognostic factors are (1) age, (2) male gender (in some studies), (3) histological type or subtype and (4) tumour extent (size, extrathyroidal invasion, lymph node and distant metastases).

There are many staging systems used for DTC (Table 1.3) with different strengths and weaknesses. The most commonly used is probably the TNM (tumour, lymph node, distant metastases). However, the idea of staging a cancer is to tailor treatment and determine prognosis. New risk stratifications are being increasingly used for tailoring more personalised treatment for low-, medium- and high-risk cancers. HiLo has questioned the need for high-dose radioiodine (RAI) ablation for low-risk cancers, and this is being followed up by the IoN trial to review whether some thyroid cancers do not require RAI at all [12]. However, these treatment options are reliant on the staging and stratification of patients into low-, medium- and high-risk groups. This can be achieved by using the histological subtype, vascular and local invasion, resection margins and cervical lymph node metastases and distant metastases to stratify the cancer in these risk groups post-operatively to guide treatment options.

Table 1.3 Staging systems used to help stratify thyroid cancer [6]

Staging system	Criteria used	Tumour
TNM	*Tumour size* (T1a <1 cm, T1b 1–2 cm, T2 2–4 cm, T3 >4 cm or minimal extrathyroidal extension, T4 invasion of surrounding structures) *Node metastases* (N1a, level VI; N1b, levels II–VII) *Distant metastases* M0–Nil, M1—present	Papillary follicular medullary
AMES	**A**ge at presentation **M**etastases Tumour **e**xtent **S**ize of primary tumour	Papillary follicular
MACIS	**M**etastases **A**ge at presentation **C**ompleteness of resection **I**nvasion **S**ize	Papillary
AGES	**A**ge at presentation **G**rade of tumour **E**xtent **S**ize	

Table 1.4 Prognosis of differentiated thyroid cancer according to stage

	Stage 1	Stage 2	Stage 3	Stage 4a	Stage 4b	Stage 4C
Follicular/papillary thyroid cancer <45 years	Any T, any N M0	Any T, any N M1				
Follicular/papillary thyroid cancer >45 years	T1, N0, M0	T2, N0, M0	T1–T3, N1a, M0 or T3, N0, M0	T1–3, N1b, M0 or T4a, any N, M0	T4b, any N, M0	Any T/N and **M1**
10-year survival %	98.5	98.8	99.0	75.9	62.5	63

The staging of differentiated thyroid cancer is strongly biased by the age of the patient using the TNM system, as the age affects outcome and prognosis. In patients under 45 years old, the prognosis is excellent even in the presence of distant metastases, and therefore, there are only two stages for patients under 45. For patients over 45 years old, there are four stages. Over the age of 45, the prognosis starts to worsen once lymph node metastases extend to the lateral cervical chain or beyond with distant metastases and creates a sudden drop in the 10-year survival to 76% from 99%. In stark comparison, anaplastic cancer has a poor prognosis with a median survival of 3–7 months and a 10–20% 1 year survival [6, 15] (Table 1.4).

Key Points

- Thyroid cancer is the most common endocrine cancer.
- There are three main types: papillary, follicular and medullary thyroid cancer.
- Rarely thyroid cancer can be anaplastic cancers which have a very poor prognosis compared with all over types of thyroid cancer.
- The European incidence of thyroid cancer has increased in the last decade by 65% in women and 69% in men.
- The prognosis of papillary and follicular thyroid cancer remains generally excellent and is currently stratified into low-, moderate- and high-risk cancers.
- Thyroid cancer most commonly presents with a lump in the neck, usually anteriorly in the thyroid, but can, less commonly, present with a lateral neck lymph node.
- Concerning clinical features associated with a thyroid nodule or goitre include a male patient, change in voice, compression symptoms, stridor, a rapidly enlarging thyroid nodule or a long-standing goitre increasing in size, a hard nodule or one fixed to the surrounding structures or the presence of cervical lymphadenopathy.
- The investigation of thyroid cancer is best performed within a specialist thyroid clinic.
- Ultrasound +/− fine needle aspiration cytology (FNAC) biopsy should be performed.
- There has also been an increase in thyroid nodules diagnosed incidentally on CT and ^{18}fluoro-deoxy-glucose positron emission tomography (FDG PET) scan.
- The Royal College of Pathologists has produced guidance for the assessment of thyroid cytology. The guidance categorises thyroid cytology as Thy1–Thy5.
- The prognosis of papillary and follicular thyroid cancer is generally very good. Even though there is a 5–20% risk of recurrence and 10–15% risk of distant metastases, only 9% of patients with DTC will die of their disease.
- The staging of differentiated thyroid cancer is strongly biased by the age of the patient using the TNM system, as the age affects outcome and prognosis.

1.4 Summary

While the incidence of thyroid cancer appears to be increasing worldwide, we are also becoming more adept at diagnosis due to an improvement in imaging and preoperative cytological diagnosis. The risk factors for thyroid cancer are multiple and include a proportion which are related to familial syndromes. On the whole, the prognosis of differentiated thyroid cancer is excellent, but new methods of stratifying the risk to a specific patient are developing to guide and individualise the treatment of thyroid cancer.

References

1. cancerresearchuk. Incidence of thyroid cancer. 2011 [cited 2014].
2. Chen AY, Jemal A, Ward EM. Increasing incidence of differentiated thyroid cancer in the United States, 1988-2005. Cancer. 2009;115(16):3801–7.
3. Aschebrook-Kilfoy B, et al. Thyroid cancer incidence patterns in the United States by histologic type, 1992-2006. Thyroid. 2011;21(2):125–34.
4. Olaleye O, et al. Increasing incidence of differentiated thyroid cancer in South East England: 1987-2006. Eur Arch Otorhinolaryngol. 2011;268(6):899–906.
5. Nose V. Familial thyroid cancer: a review. Mod Pathol. 2011;24(Suppl 2):S19–33.
6. Perros P, et al. Guidelines for the management of thyroid cancer. Clin Endocrinol (Oxf). 2014;81(Suppl 1):–1, 122.
7. Hegedus L, Bonnema SJ, Bennedbaek FN. Management of simple nodular goiter: current status and future perspectives. Endocr Rev. 2003;24(1):102–32.
8. Frates MC, et al. Management of thyroid nodules detected at US: Society of Radiologists in Ultrasound consensus conference statement. Radiology. 2005;237(3):794–800.
9. Kim EK, et al. New sonographic criteria for recommending fine-needle aspiration biopsy of nonpalpable solid nodules of the thyroid. AJR Am J Roentgenol. 2002;178(3):687–91.
10. Gharib H, et al. American Association of Clinical Endocrinologists and Associazione Medici Endocrinologi medical guidelines for clinical practice for the diagnosis and management of thyroid nodules. Endocr Pract. 2006;12(1):63–102.
11. Ahn SS, et al. Biopsy of thyroid nodules: comparison of three sets of guidelines. AJR Am J Roentgenol. 2010;194(1):31–7.
12. Park JM, Choi Y, Kwag HJ. Partially cystic thyroid nodules: ultrasound findings of malignancy. Korean J Radiol. 2012;13(5):530–5.
13. Soelberg KK, et al. Risk of malignancy in thyroid incidentalomas detected by 18F-fluorodeoxyglucose positron emission tomography: a systematic review. Thyroid. 2012;22(9):918–25.
14. www.rcpath, T.R.C.o.P. Guidance on the reporting of thyroid cytology specimens. 2009.
15. Untch BR, Olson JA Jr. Anaplastic thyroid carcinoma, thyroid lymphoma, and metastasis to thyroid. Surg Oncol Clin N Am. 2006;15(3):661–79, x.

Thyroid Cancer Pathology

Susannah L. Shore

Contents

2.1	Papillary Cancer	9
2.2	Follicular Variant Papillary Carcinoma	10
2.3	Papillary Microcarcinoma	10
2.4	Follicular Cancer	10
2.5	Oncocytic (Hurthle Cell) Tumours	11
2.6	Poorly Differentiated Thyroid Cancer	11
2.7	Anaplastic Cancer	12
References		13

2.1 Papillary Cancer

Papillary cancer is the most common thyroid malignancy (85%). It most commonly occurs in women of the third to fifth decade. However, it also occurs in children. Papillary cancer is importantly associated with radiation exposure confirmed by the epidemic of thyroid cancer in children and babies following the Chernobyl nuclear power station disaster [1, 2]. It is derived from the follicular epithelium and has a papillary growth pattern with psammoma bodies and characteristic nuclear changes that can be diagnosed on cytology. These include Orphan Annie nuclei, intranuclear inclusions of cytoplasm and nuclear grooves although inclusions and nuclear grooves can be seen in Hashimoto's disease [3]. Papillary cancers invade the lymphatics resulting in multifocality and lymph node metastases. Venous invasion is less commonly seen (5–7%) causing lung and bone metastases [4]. There are many

S.L. Shore
Royal Liverpool and Broadgreen University Hospitals NHS Trust, Liverpool, UK
e-mail: Susannah.shore@rlbuht.nhs.uk

variants to the classic papillary cancer, some of which are known to have more aggressive behaviour including tall cell variant, columnar cell variant and diffuse sclerotic type and in stratifications are usually categorised into high-risk groups. There are two more categories that require further discussion.

2.2 Follicular Variant Papillary Carcinoma

A tumour showing follicular architecture with papillary thyroid nuclear appearances. There are three main types with different behaviours:

1. *Nonencapsulated or infiltrative type* which behaves clinically like a classical papillary thyroid cancer.
2. *Encapsulated lesions* have more similarities with follicular neoplasm, and the behaviour depends more on whether the lesion demonstrates capsular and vascular invasion. *Encapsulated non-invasive lesions* have a very low risk of recurrence or metastases [5]. *Encapsulated invasive lesions* in the presence of vascular invasion behave as a low-grade malignancy.
3. *Diffuse/aggressive/multinodular* is a rare tumour more commonly found in young patients and has a more aggressive nature.

2.3 Papillary Microcarcinoma

Papillary microcarcinoma is a relatively recently described phenomenon and is thought to be in part responsible for the increasing incidence of thyroid cancer. A microcarcinoma is described as a carcinoma less than 10 mm. Usually, these are micropapillary carcinomas but can more unusually be follicular or medullary carcinomas. The prognosis is usually excellent with a mortality of 0.34% [6]. However, these microcarcinomas can have lymph node metastases 12–50% [5] and sometimes patients present with them. Risk factors for recurrence include clinical (not incidental) presentation, multifocality and lymph node metastases at diagnosis [6]. Other factors include PET-positive lesions, extrathyroidal extension and poorly differentiated component [5]. The treatment of papillary microcarcinoma with no adverse features should be limited to a hemithyroidectomy and GP follow-up; however, those microcarcinomas with any adverse features should be risk stratified and discussed at MDT.

2.4 Follicular Cancer

A follicular carcinoma is from follicular epithelial cell origin with evidence of capsular (and/or vascular) invasion but without nuclear changes characteristic of papillary thyroid cancer. It represents 10–20% of thyroid cancers and is unusual in childhood. Follicular carcinomas have a slightly poorer prognosis than papillary thyroid cancers. Metastatic spread is haematogenous most commonly to the lung and bone. As the carcinoma is defined by capsular invasion, the diagnosis cannot be made by cytological assessment from a FNAC (fine needle aspiration cytology), nor can a malignant lesion be excluded intraoperatively with a frozen section assessment as the lesion must be extensively sampled to exclude a potential single focus of capsular invasion. The extent of capsular invasion and the presence and the multifocality of vascular invasion increase the risk of metastases and confer a poorer prognosis. As these two factors tend to change the prognosis of follicular carcinomas, this category is divided into two types of follicular cancer, which can vary widely in appearance and prognosis:

1. *Minimally invasive follicular carcinoma*
   Minimally invasive follicular carcinoma is a single encapsulated nodule that has only focal microscopic and/or vascular invasion. Tumours with *capsular invasion only* have a minimal risk of metastases. Tumours with *capsular and vascular invasion* may develop blood-borne metastases. There is some evidence that four or more foci of vascular invasion equate to a worsened prognosis [7].
2. *Widely invasive follicular carcinoma*
   These tumours have a worse prognosis and are defined by the presence of extensive microscopic invasion of thyroid parenchyma, capsule or extratumoural vessels or gross macroscopic tumour invasion. These tumours are more aggressive with a poorer prognosis especially when associated with gross invasion (macroscopic extrathyroidal extension (EXE)) as opposed to microscopic EXE [5, 7].

2.5 Oncocytic (Hurthle Cell) Tumours

Oncocytic or Hurthle cell change can occur in any thyroid tumour type but is more commonly associated with follicular carcinomas. Diagnostic criteria are the same, but the prognosis for oncocytic tumours is worse for comparative stage mainly as a result of the oncocytic carcinoma showing poor radioiodine uptake. Oncocytic cells can be found in ordinary follicular lesions, so this tumour requires 75% oncocytic cell change regardless of histological pattern [7].

2.6 Poorly Differentiated Thyroid Cancer

This group of cancers show an intermediate degree of differentiation between anaplastic carcinomas and follicular epithelial-derived cancers and carry a poorer prognosis. Cells may demonstrate necrosis and increased mitotic counts. Insular carcinomas fall into this category. Cells may express thyroglobulin and may respond to radioiodine therapy. Fifty per cent of tumour cells must be of this type to diagnose a poorly differentiated thyroid cancer; however, smaller foci may also confer a prognostic implication [5, 7].

2.7 Anaplastic Cancer

Anaplastic carcinoma is diagnosed in the presence of undifferentiated (anaplastic) tumour. These tumours are aggressive and generally have a short clinical course and poor prognosis. They most commonly occur in women over the age of 65. It can develop on a background of DTC (differentiated thyroid cancer), and multiple mutations have been reported (p53, BRAF, RAS, PTEN). Tumour growth is usually rapid, and the majority arises in a pre-existing goitre. At presentation, the majority will already have advanced disease with tracheal, oesophageal or vascular involvement and therefore beyond surgical curative resection. One year survival is 10–20% [8], and outcome relies on stage at presentation and multimodal treatment [7].

> **Key Points**
>
> - Papillary cancer is the most common thyroid malignancy (85%). It most commonly occurs in women of the third to fifth decade.
>
> - Papillary cancer is derived from follicular epithelium and has a papillary growth pattern with psammoma bodies and characteristic nuclear changes that can be diagnosed on cytology.
>
> - Papillary cancers invade the lymphatics resulting in multifocality and lymph node metastases.
>
> - A follicular carcinoma is from follicular epithelial cell origin with evidence of capsular (and/or vascular) invasion but without nuclear changes characteristic of papillary thyroid cancer.
>
> - Follicular carcinoma represents 10–20% of thyroid cancers and is unusual in childhood. Follicular carcinomas have a slightly poorer prognosis than papillary thyroid cancers.
>
> - Metastatic spread from follicular carcinoma is haematogenous most commonly to the lung and bone (as the carcinoma is defined by capsular invasion, the diagnosis cannot be made by cytological assessment from a FNAC).
>
> - The extent of capsular invasion and the presence and the multifocality of vascular invasion increase the risk of metastases and confer a poorer prognosis.
>
> - Oncocytic or Hurthle cell change can occur in any thyroid tumour type but is more commonly associated with follicular carcinomas.
>
> - Poorly differentiated thyroid cancer carries a poor prognosis.
>
> - Anaplastic carcinoma is diagnosed in the presence of undifferentiated (anaplastic) tumour. These tumours are aggressive and generally have a short clinical course and poor prognosis.

References

1. Becker DV, et al. Childhood thyroid cancer following the Chernobyl accident: a status report. Endocrinol Metab Clin North Am. 1996;25(1):197–211.
2. Tuttle RM, Becker DV. The Chernobyl accident and its consequences: update at the millennium. Semin Nucl Med. 2000;30(2):133–40.
3. LiVolsi VA. Papillary thyroid carcinoma: an update. Mod Pathol. 2011;24(Suppl 2):S1–9.
4. Hoie J, et al. Distant metastases in papillary thyroid cancer. A review of 91 patients. Cancer. 1988;61(1):1–6.
5. Perros P, et al. Guidelines for the management of thyroid cancer. Clin Endocrinol (Oxf). 2014;81(Suppl 1):1–122.
6. Roti E, et al. Thyroid papillary microcarcinoma: a descriptive and meta-analysis study. Eur J Endocrinol. 2008;159(6):659–73.
7. Stephenson TJ, Johnson S. Dataset for thyroid cancer histopathology reports. London: Royal College of Pathologists; 2014.
8. Kebebew E. Anaplastic thyroid carcinoma: rare, fatal and neglected. Surgery. 2012;152:1088–9.

Management of Thyroid Cancer

3

M.P. Rowland, A.J. Waghorn, and S. Vinjamuri

Contents

3.1	Introduction	16
3.2	Diagnosis and Perioperative Assessment	16
3.3	Management of Differentiated Thyroid Cancer: Based on Histological Type	16
	3.3.1 Differentiated Thyroid Cancers (DTCs) >1 cm (Papillary and Follicular Thyroid Cancer)	16
	3.3.2 Micro-papillary Carcinomas (<1 cm)	17
	3.3.3 Follicular Thyroid Cancers	17
	3.3.4 Hurthle (Oncocytic) Cell-Variant Follicular Tumours	17
3.4	Central and Lateral Neck Lymph Node Dissections in DTC	18
3.5	Adjuvant Treatments in Differentiated Thyroid Cancer	18
	3.5.1 Radioiodine Remnant Ablation (RRA) and Therapy for Differentiated Thyroid Cancer	18
3.6	Post-ablation Follow-Up in DTC	19
3.7	External Beam Radiotherapy (EBRT)	19
3.8	Management of Rare Thyroid Malignancies	20
	3.8.1 Medullary Thyroid Cancer (MTC)	20
	3.8.2 Surgery	20
	3.8.3 Micro-MTC (<5 mm) and At-Risk Individuals	20
	3.8.4 Adjuvant Therapies for MTC	21
3.9	Thyroid Lymphoma	21
3.10	Anaplastic Thyroid Cancer	21
References		23

M.P. Rowland (✉) • A.J. Waghorn
Department of Surgery, Royal Liverpool University Hospital, Liverpool, UK
e-mail: Alison.waghorn@rlbuht.nhs.uk

S. Vinjamuri
Department of Nuclear Medicine, Royal Liverpool and Broadgreen University Hospitals NHS Trust, Liverpool, UK

© Springer International Publishing AG, part of Springer Nature 2018
S. Vinjamuri (ed.), *PET/CT in Thyroid Cancer*, Clinicians' Guides to Radionuclide Hybrid Imaging, https://doi.org/10.1007/978-3-319-71846-0_3

3.1 Introduction

Thyroid cancer treatment encompassed a heterogeneous group of malignancies with both surgical and adjuvant medical aspects to its management. This chapter reviews the current UK management practice for differentiated thyroid cancer (DTC) followed by less commonly occurring thyroid malignancies.

Most thyroid malignancies have an extremely good prognosis; however, this good prognosis can only be achieved and maintained by high-quality diagnosis and treatments overseen by an experienced multidisciplinary team (MDT). The most recent 2014 British Thyroid Association (BTA) guidelines, fully endorsed by the British Association of Endocrine and Thyroid Surgeons (BAETS), aim to promote the high-quality evidence-based practice, reducing variability of treatment and patient-centred approach [1]. Within the guidance is an increasing emphasis on less aggressive surgical resections and lymph node dissections for good-prognosis disease and a more structured and evidence-based use of adjuvant treatments. This chapter will review the essential evidence-based thyroid cancer practice in the UK.

3.2 Diagnosis and Perioperative Assessment

Urgent referrals for possible thyroid cancer should be managed in line with the Department of Health guidelines for possible malignancy, with prompt assessment by a member of the thyroid MDT [2]. Clinical assessment included relevant family history of thyroid cancer and biochemical assessment of the endocrine system; assessment of thyroid nodules should involve the use of ultrasound (US) with fine needle aspiration cytology (FNAC) if appropriate [3]. Standardised grading systems are in place for both US and cytological reporting are now strongly encouraged [4, 5]. Results and use of staging investigation should be discussed at a head and neck or dedicated thyroid MDT and the patient informed of the diagnosis with support of a specialist nurse and written materials [6]. The majority of thyroid cancers will be appropriate for surgical resection; however, in some patients with other complex health problems or other synchronous malignancies, a thyroid resection may not be the priority or required; an MDT documentation of this is essential.

3.3 Management of Differentiated Thyroid Cancer: Based on Histological Type

3.3.1 Differentiated Thyroid Cancers (DTCs) >1 cm (Papillary and Follicular Thyroid Cancer)

Nodules that are suspicious, but not diagnosed, as a thyroid cancer preoperatively should be managed with a diagnostic hemithyroidectomy [7]; a delayed completion thyroidectomy +/− lymph node dissection may be required following discussion of the histology. Intraoperative frozen section may be appropriate to facilitate one-stage operation for a mass that is highly likely to be malignant, but it has been impossible to confirm it preoperatively [8].

BTA guidelines (2014) recommend total thyroidectomy for patients with tumours greater than 4 cm in diameter or tumours of any size in association with any of the following characteristics: *multifocal disease, extra-thyroidal spread (pT3 and pT4a), familial disease and those with clinically or radiologically involved nodes and/or distant metastases* [9]. At the time of thyroidectomy, the surgeon should be alert to abnormal lymph nodes (not detected preoperatively) and undertake bilateral central neck dissection with total thyroidectomy if the nodes are positive on frozen section; what unilateral central dissection does is not an appropriate way to stage the nodal status of the neck and is discouraged [10, 11]. Patients not falling into the above groups are likely to be appropriately treated with a hemithyroidectomy without lymph node dissection.

3.3.2 Micro-papillary Carcinomas (<1 cm)

Classical papillary microcarcinoma (<1 cm) is a common incidental finding on hemithyroidectomy or finding on US scans; following hemithyroidectomy, further surgery is not indicated if it is a single focus and has no other risk features identified [12]. If the microcarcinoma is multifocal, invading thyroid capsule or found within a family who has papillary carcinoma, then further surgery should be considered.

3.3.3 Follicular Thyroid Cancers

Differentiated follicular-type tumours most commonly present as a solitary lesion that on histology is shown to be a minimally invasive follicular lesion with widely invasive follicular tumours tending to behave as a more aggressive thyroid cancer, with higher incidence of distant metastatic disease from haematogenous spread often with macroscopic invasion into local blood vessels on histology [13]. Follicular thyroid cancer rarely metastasises to lymph nodes (1–8% of follicular cancer [14]) limiting the need for lymph node dissection in the majority of cases.

Patients with tumours larger than 4 cm should be treated with a total thyroidectomy. Patients with tumours <4 cm in the absence of other adverse risk factors (age >45, widely invasive, lymph node or distant metastases, angio-invasion) appear to have excellent prognosis [15]; hemithyroidectomy alone should be considered by the MDT.

3.3.4 Hurthle (Oncocytic) Cell-Variant Follicular Tumours

Hurthle cell is appreciated to have a worse prognosis compared with follicular thyroid cancer [16] and other types of DTC, which may partly reflect less cellular differentiation resulting in lack of ability to take up radioiodine. Total thyroidectomy is recommended for oncocytic (Hurthle cell) carcinomas >1 cm in diameter; therapeutic lymph node dissection should be performed in patients with clinical/radiological evidence of lymph node involvement and pathological confirmation of metastasis as with other differentiated thyroid cancers [17].

3.4 Central and Lateral Neck Lymph Node Dissections in DTC

Central lymph node dissections (level VI +/− VII) in patients with papillary cancer >1 cm are no longer recommended as routine; a central neck dissection without clinical or radiological evidence of lymph node involvement can be considered in those who have all of the following characteristics: non-classical-type PTC, age >45 years, multifocal tumour, tumour >4 cm and extra-thyroidal extension on ultrasound [18, 19].

In patients who present with overt metastatic disease in the lateral neck, 80% will be identified to have central compartment nodal disease, either clinically or radiologically [20]. All those who present with lateral neck disease should have central and lateral neck dissections (levels IIa–Vb), but there is no longer an indication for prophylactic lateral neck lymph node dissection in patients with no evidence of central compartment lymph node metastases [15].

3.5 Adjuvant Treatments in Differentiated Thyroid Cancer

3.5.1 Radioiodine Remnant Ablation (RRA) and Therapy for Differentiated Thyroid Cancer

Radioiodine remnant ablation (RRA) and ^{131}I therapy should be supervised by a clinical oncologist or nuclear medicine physician with expertise and an interest in management of DTC: The physician should be a core member of a thyroid cancer MDT [21]. Tumours >4 cm or any tumour (independent of size) with extra-thyroidal extension (pT3 and pT4) or distant metastases should be advised to *receive* RRA; any tumour <1 cm, unifocal or multifocal, histologically classical papillary or follicular variant (with no invasion of the thyroid capsule) or minimally invasive follicular without angio-invasion should be advised *against* receiving RRA [22]. For those tumours between 1 and 4 cm, the data is equivocal, and cases should be discussed on an individual basis or be entered into a trial [22].

Current recommendations in the BTA guidelines (2014) advise that recombinant TSH (rbTSH) is the recommended method of preparation for RRA in patients with the following characteristics: *pT1–pT3, p N0 or NX or N1 and M0 and R0 (no microscopic residual disease)* [22]. In disease with a poorer prognosis, thyroxine withdrawal should be considered, but certain patients do not tolerate this, e.g. depressive patients and patients with multiple co-morbidities [22]. If a patient undergoes hormone withdrawal prior to I^{131} therapy, levothyroxine should be restarted when the patient is discharged following their I^{131} therapy. Those patients who will likely undergo thyroid hormone withdrawal should be placed on liothyronine (T3) as soon as possible after surgery. RRA is usually

Table 3.1 Reproduction of Table 2.3 BTA: Management of Thyroid Cancer 2014 guidance

Excellent response	Indeterminate response	Incomplete response
All the following	Any of the following	Any of the following
• Suppressed and stimulated Tg <1 µg/L[a]	• Suppressed Tg <1 µg/L[a] and stimulated Tg ≥1 and <10 µg/L[a]	• Suppressed Tg ≥1 µg/L[a] or stimulated Tg <10 µg/L[a]
		• Rising Tg values
• Neck US without evidence of disease	• Neck US with nonspecific changes or stable sub centimetre lymph nodes	• Persistent or newly identified disease on cross-sectional and/or nuclear medicine imaging
• Cross-sectional and/or nuclear medicine imaging negative (if performed)	• Cross-sectional and/or nuclear medicine imaging with nonspecific changes» although not completely normal	
Low risk	Intermediate risk	High risk

[a]Assumes absence of interference in the Tg assay

delivered over 4 weeks from surgery, when all the patient's own thyroxine has been excreted or degraded. Pregnancy must be excluded before RRA or ^{131}I therapy is administered and advised against for at least 8 months after; breast-feeding must be discontinued at least 8 weeks before RRA or ^{131}I therapy to avoid breast radiation [22].

Patients who have undergone a total thyroidectomy and RRA should undergo dynamic risk stratification (DRS). DRS involves the tailoring of further imaging and specific levels/length of TSH suppression depending on an individual's response to treatment. TSH suppression is created by titrating up the levothyroxine dose but avoiding frank hyperthyroidism (see Table 3.1 for current guidance for dynamic risk stratification after RRA or ^{131}I therapy).

3.6 Post-ablation Follow-Up in DTC

Post-ablation scan should be performed after ^{131}I when residual activity levels permit satisfactory imaging (2–10 days) with patients continuing on levothyroxine (T4), rather than liothyronine (T3) between the RRA and the post-ablation scans [23]. The new recommendation is for stimulated thyroglobulin (Tg) and ultrasound of the neck rather than routine diagnostic ^{131}I whole body scanning, between 9 and 12 months post RRA. In cases where the measurement of serum-Tg is unreliable, and where ^{131}I uptake was visualised beyond the thyroid bed and neck in the post-ablation scan a diagnostic whole body scan with ^{123}I or ^{131}I [23]; SPECT-CT may be combined to give better anatomical localisation of possible recurrence.

3.7 External Beam Radiotherapy (EBRT)

External beam radiotherapy is rarely used in well –differentiated thyroid cancer, the current guidance stating the indication for consideration of adjuvant EBRT is for patients with a high risk of recurrence/progression with: *"a) gross evidence of local tumour invasion at surgery with significant macroscopic residual disease or b) residual or recurrent tumour that fails to concentrate radioiodine"* [24] i.e. locoregional disease where further surgery or radioiodine is ineffective or impractical. Metastatic bone disease can often be treated with both ^{131}I and external beam radiotherapy and occasionally surgical fixation or resection.

3.8 Management of Rare Thyroid Malignancies

3.8.1 Medullary Thyroid Cancer (MTC)

MTC is a rare thyroid cancer (3% of adult thyroid cancers [25]) but behaves more aggressively compared to DTCs. In almost all cases, it is associated with elevated serum calcitonin and often CEA protein [25] as well. All patients with or at risk of MTC should be referred for investigation and/or treatment with a thyroid cancer specialist, where a comprehensive family history should be taken to include first-/second-degree relatives to search for features of MEN 2 (e.g. MTC, phaeochromocytoma, hyperparathyroidism) and familial MTC [25]. All MTC should have biochemical screening for phaeochromocytoma before undergoing surgical resection. Up to 25% of patients will have a genetic origin and all should be offered genetic analysis.

3.8.2 Surgery

All patients with established MTC should undergo a minimum of total thyroidectomy and central neck dissection (levels VI and VII); if central neck dissection is shown to have lymph node metastases, then further lateral neck dissection should be considered [26]. Ipsilateral lateral neck dissection is recommended if there are central neck metastases (70% of those with central metastases have lateral neck metastases). Preoperative imaging is not a good predictor of nodal metastases in MTC. In view of the fact that this cancer is managed with a philosophy of curative resection or continued 'de-bulking' strategy, in all patients, surgical resection is considered the best treatment, and disease in the mediastinum should be considered for surgery using sternotomy if needed. In patients with distant metastases, surgery should be considered to prevent subsequent compromise of the trachea, oesophagus and recurrent laryngeal nerves. During a resection, these structures should ideally be preserved where possible with a plan to perform redo resection if further recurrence occurs.

3.8.3 Micro-MTC (<5 mm) and At-Risk Individuals

Incidental, sporadic (RET negative) and unifocal micro-MTCs can be treated with hemithyroidectomy; however, up to 20% of patients may have nodal metastases [26]. Calcitonin and CEA levels should be used to monitor for recurrence and predict the need for further surgery.

Prophylactic surgery should be offered to disease-free carriers of germ line RET mutations, identified by genetic screening. The timing of such surgery will depend on the genotype and age of the patient [26].

3.8.4 Adjuvant Therapies for MTC

Radioiodine ablation is not an option for MTC, and routine external beam radiotherapy (EBRT) is not recommended; EBRT should only be considered once optimal surgery has been performed, and there is a significant risk of local recurrent disease (e.g. macroscopic residual disease or microscopic residual disease) on a background of large volume disease [27].

Chemotherapy is rarely used with doxorubicin felt to produce symptomatic response in less than 30% of cases, and most are partial and of short duration.

Radioisotope treatment shows some promise for this disease; there are data showing response in patients with progressive disease for ^{90}yttrium-DOTATOC for patients with uptake on a diagnostic ^{111}In-octreotide scan. ^{131}I MIBG and ^{90}Y/^{177}Lu-labelled peptides have limited evidence to support their use although one study did show symptom palliation in 61% of MTC patients with ^{131}I MIBG [28].

Overall increased survival has been reported with pre-targeted radio-immunotherapy using bio-specific monoclonal anti-CEA antibodies and a ^{131}I-labelled bivalent hapten for patients with metastatic progressive MTC with survival of 110 months versus 61 months [29].

3.9 Thyroid Lymphoma

This is a tumour almost always associated with autoimmune thyroiditis with elevated TPO antibodies; it often involves the whole thyroid gland. It is usually treated with chemo +/− radiotherapy under the care of a haematologist. Core biopsy or open incision biopsy (rather than FNAC) will be needed to confirm diagnosis; rarely a lymphoma can be found in a specific nodule (MALT lymphoma); a hemithyroidectomy may be sufficient treatment. Each individual needs to be discussed at appropriate MDTs.

3.10 Anaplastic Thyroid Cancer

This tumour presents with a fast-growing and invasive nature; by the time the tumour presents, it is usually irresectable and difficult to treat. Initial assessment should focus in identifying the small proportion of patients with localised disease and good performance status that may benefit from surgical resection and other adjuvant therapies. Surgical de-bulking of anaplastic thyroid cancer is not advised for those tumours that are irresectable; chemo-radiotherapy may be considered [30], but in many this makes little difference to prognosis.

Key Points

Well-Differentiated Papillary Thyroid Cancer
- Total thyroidectomy is the resection of choice for tumours greater than 4 cm in diameter; many smaller tumours can be managed by hemithyroidectomy.

- Papillary microcarcinoma is a common incidental finding on hemithyroidectomy, and further surgery is not indicated if it is unifocal and has no other risk features.

- Avoid central neck dissection (level VI +/− VII) without clinical or radiological evidence of lymph node involvement for the majority of patients.

- Patients with positive central lymph nodes should undergo total thyroidectomy and bilateral level VI dissection.

- All those patients who present with lateral neck disease should have central and lateral neck dissections (levels IIa–Vb) along with a total thyroidectomy.

Follicular Thyroid Cancer
- Tumours with greater than 4 cm tumour should be treated with a total thyroidectomy.

- Patients with tumours <4 cm in the absence of other adverse risk factors often only require hemithyroidectomy.

Hurthle Cell Follicular Tumours
- Total thyroidectomy is recommended for oncocytic (Hurthle cell) carcinomas >1 cm in diameter with therapeutic lymph node dissection performed in patients with clinical/radiological evidence of lymph node involvement and pathological confirmation of metastasis.

Radioiodine Remnant Ablation (RRA)
- Any tumour >4 cm or any tumour (independent of size) with gross extrathyroidal extension (pT4) or distant metastases should be advised to receive RRA.

- Patients who have undergone a total thyroidectomy and RRA should undergo dynamic risk stratification to determine levels and length of TSH suppression.

- External beam radiotherapy is rarely used in well-differentiated thyroid cancer.

Medullary Thyroid Cancer (MTC)
- All patients with or at risk of MTC should be referred for investigation/surgical treatment centre.

- All patients with established MTC (>1 cm) should undergo a minimum of total thyroidectomy and central neck dissection (levels VI and VII).

- Prophylactic surgery should be offered to disease-free carriers of germ line RET mutations.

- New molecular therapies may hold promise for management of recurrent disease.

Thyroid Lymphoma
- Lymphoma involves the whole thyroid gland and is treated with chemo +/− radiotherapy.

- A core biopsy or open incision biopsy is needed to confirm diagnosis.

Anaplastic Thyroid Cancer
- Surgical de-bulking of anaplastic thyroid cancer is not advised.

- For irresectable tumours, chemo-radiotherapy treatment may assist in palliation.

References

1. Perros P, Boelaert K, Colley S, et al. Guidelines for the management of thyroid cancer. Clin Endocrinol (Oxf). 2014;81:–1, 122.
2. Department of Health. (2006) Cancer Waiting Times: A Guide (Version 5). London: DH. www.dh.gov.uk/en/Publicationsandstatistics/Publications/PublicationsPolicyAndGuidance/DH_06306761.
3. Hambly NM, Gonen M, Gerst SR. Implementation of Evidence-based guidelines for thyroid nodule biopsy: a model for establishment of practice standards. Am J Roentgenol. 2011;196:655–60.
4. Perros P, Boelaert K, Colley S, et al. Guidelines for the management of thyroid cancer—Chapter 4 Ultrasound assessment of thyroid nodules. Clin Endocrinol (Oxf). 2014;81:14–8.
5. Perros P, Boelaert K, Colley S, et al. Guidelines for the management of thyroid cancer—Chapter 5 Fine-Needle aspiration cytology. Clin Endocrinol (Oxf). 2014;81:19–20.
6. Perros P, Boelaert K, Colley S, et al. Guidelines for the management of thyroid cancer—Chapter 3 Presentation, diagnosis and referral. Clin Endocrinol (Oxf). 2014;81:10–1.
7. Perros P, Boelaert K, Colley S, et al. Guidelines for the management of thyroid cancer—Chapter 7.5 Diagnostic thyroid surgery. Clin Endocrinol (Oxf). 2014;81:26.
8. Seningen JL, Nassar A, Henry MR. Correlation of thyroid nodule fine-needle aspiration cytology with corresponding histology at Mayo Clinic, 2001-2007: an institutional experience of 1,945 cases. Diagn Cytopathol. 2012;40(Suppl. 1):E27–32.
9. Perros P, Boelaert K, Colley S, et al. Guidelines for the management of thyroid cancer—Chapter 7.6 Therapeutic surgery for thyroid cancer. Clin Endocrinol (Oxf). 2014;81:27.
10. Hart DM, Leboulleux S, Al Ghuzlan A, et al. Optimization of staging of the neck with prophylactic central and lateral neck dissection for papillary thyroid carcinoma. Ann Surg. 2012;255:777–83.
11. Lang BH, Wong KP, Wan KY, et al. Impact of routine unilateral central neck dissection on preablative and postablative stimulated thyroglobulin levels after total thyroidectomy in papillary thyroid carcinoma. Ann Surg Oncol. 2012;19:60–7.
12. Perros P, Boelaert K, Colley S, et al. Guidelines for the management of thyroid cancer—Chapter 8.3 Management of papillary microcarcinoma. Clin Endocrinol (Oxf). 2014;81:33.

13. Lang W, Choritz H, Hundeshagen H. Risk factors in follicular thyroid carcinomas. A retrospective follow-up study covering a 14-year period with emphasis on morphological findings. Am J Surg Pathol. 1986;10:246–55.
14. Nagar S, Aschebrook-Kilfoy B, Kaplan EL, et al. Hurthle cell carcinoma: an update on survival over the last 35 years. Surgery. 2013;154:1263–71.
15. Perros P, Boelaert K, Colley S, et al. Guidelines for the management of thyroid cancer—Chapter 7.6 Therapeutic surgery for thyroid cancer. Clin Endocrinol (Oxf). 2014;81:28.
16. Kushchayeva Y, Duh QY, Kebebew E, et al. Comparison of clinical characteristics at diagnosis and during follow-up in 118 patients with Hurthle cell or follicular thyroid cancer. Am J Surg. 2008;195:457–62.
17. Perros P, Boelaert K, Colley S, et al. Guidelines for the management of thyroid cancer—Chapter 7.8 Therapeutic surgery for thyroid cancer. Clin Endocrinol (Oxf). 2014;81:29.
18. Baek SK, Jung KY, Kang SM, et al. Clinical risk factors associated with cervical lymph node recurrence in papillary thyroid carcinoma. Thyroid. 2010;20:147–52.
19. Ito Y, Kudo T, Kobayashi K, et al. Prognostic factors for recurrence of papillary thyroid carcinoma in the lymph nodes, lung, and bone: analysis of 5,768 patients with average 10-year follow-up. World J Surg. 2012;36:1274–8.
20. Farrag T, Lin F, Brownlee N, et al. Is routine dissection of level II-B and V-A necessary in patients with papillary thyroid cancer undergoing lateral neck dissection for FNA-confirmed metastases in other levels. World J Surg. 2009;33:1680–3.
21. Perros P, Boelaert K, Colley S, et al. Guidelines for the management of thyroid cancer—Chapter 9 Radioiodine remnant ablation and therapy for differentiated thyroid cancer. Clin Endocrinol (Oxf). 2014;81:37.
22. Perros P, Boelaert K, Colley S, et al. Guidelines for the management of thyroid cancer—Chapter 9 Radioiodine remnant ablation and therapy for differentiated thyroid cancer. Clin Endocrinol (Oxf). 2014;81:38.
23. Perros P, Boelaert K, Colley S, et al. Guidelines for the management of thyroid cancer—Chapter 9.7 Radioiodine remnant ablation and therapy for differentiated thyroid cancer. Clin Endocrinol (Oxf). 2014;81:42.
24. Perros P, Boelaert K, Colley S, et al. Guidelines for the management of thyroid cancer—Chapter 10.1. External beam radiotherapy for differentiated thyroid cancer. Clin Endocrinol (Oxf). 2014;81:46.
25. Perros P, Boelaert K, Colley S, et al. Guidelines for the management of thyroid cancer—Chapter 17. Medullary thyroid cancer. Clin Endocrinol (Oxf). 2014;81:69.
26. Perros P, Boelaert K, Colley S, et al. Guidelines for the management of thyroid cancer—Chapter 17.3. Medullary thyroid cancer. Clin Endocrinol (Oxf). 2014;81:70.
27. Fife KM, Bower M, Harmer C. Medullary thyroid cancer: the role of radiotherapy in local control. Eur J Surg Oncol. 1996;22:588–91.
28. Iten F, Müller B, Schindler C, et al. Response to [90Yttrium-DOTA]-TOC treatment is associated with long-term survival benefit in metastasized medullary thyroid cancer: a phase II clinical trial. Clin Cancer Res. 2007;13(Pt 1):6696–702.
29. Kraeber-Bodéré F, Rousseau C, Bodet-Milin C, et al. Targeting, toxicity, and efficacy of 2-step, pretargeted radioimmunotherapy using a chimeric bispecific antibody and 131I-labeled bivalent hapten in a phase I optimization clinical trial. J Nucl Med. 2006;47:247–55.
30. Perros P, Boelaert K, Colley S, et al. Guidelines for the management of thyroid cancer—Chapter 18. Anaplastic thyroid cancer. Clin Endocrinol (Oxf). 2014;81:79–80.

Radiological Imaging in Thyroid Cancer

Rashika Fernando

Contents

4.1	Introduction	25
4.2	Primary Diagnosis	26
4.3	Pathological Types of Malignant Thyroid Nodules	26
	4.3.1 Differentiating Benign from Malignant Thyroid Nodules on USS	26
4.4	Ultrasound Pitfalls	27
4.5	Mixed Solid Cystic Lesions	27
4.6	FNAC of Thyroid Lesions	27
4.7	Staging	28
4.8	Primary Tumour Staging	28
4.9	Nodal Staging	28
4.10	Distant Metastases	29
4.11	Surveillance	29
References		31

4.1 Introduction

Partly as a result of the subclinical detection with imaging, the incidence of thyroid cancer is increasing [1]. Thyroid lesions are commonly encountered in diagnostic radiology with reported incidence of 30–70% on ultrasound [2]. Less than 7% of thyroid nodules are malignant, but it is vital that they are accurately diagnosed [3]. The most important factor in managing a thyroid nodule is differentiating a benign

R. Fernando
Royal Liverpool and Broadgreen University Hospitals NHS Trust, London, UK
e-mail: Rashika.fernando@rlbuht.nhs.uk

© Springer International Publishing AG, part of Springer Nature 2018
S. Vinjamuri (ed.), *PET/CT in Thyroid Cancer*, Clinicians' Guides to Radionuclide Hybrid Imaging, https://doi.org/10.1007/978-3-319-71846-0_4

lesion from a malignant nodule or identifying a malignant nodule in the setting of a multinodular goitre. This helps identify patients who will require early aggressive treatment and avoid unnecessary investigation and surgery in the majority who have a benign lesion. Given its high sensitivity, ultrasound is the most commonly used modality in the primary diagnosis and assessment of the thyroid. In contrast, CT and MRI are inferior in the detection and characterisation of thyroid nodules. The main role of these modalities is to assess for extrathyroidal tumour extension, nodal disease and distant metastases.

4.2 Primary Diagnosis

The main roles of ultrasound are the initial detection of the thyroid nodule, differentiating the majority benign nodules from malignant thyroid nodules, helping in the decision-making as to which thyroid nodules to perform fine needle aspiration cytology (FNAC)/biopsy on, and finally aiding in guiding FNAC [4].

Thyroid cancer may have variable imaging characteristics on ultrasound, and it may be difficult to differentiate from a benign nodule. Lesions can remain of indeterminate nature even after FNAC/core biopsy [5]. However, given the high sensitivity of ultrasound, the British Thyroid Society recommends that ultrasound should be performed by a competent operator in all patients assessed for possible thyroid malignancy [6].

4.3 Pathological Types of Malignant Thyroid Nodules

The main histopathological types of thyroid cancer are papillary (75%), follicular (10%—hurtle cell is a more aggressive variant of follicular), medullary (5%) and anaplastic (<5%). Lymphoma (<5%) and metastases (predominantly lung, breast and renal) are also rare, as is sarcoma [7].

4.3.1 Differentiating Benign from Malignant Thyroid Nodules on USS

4.3.1.1 Benign Nodules
- Purely cystic nodule [8, 9]
- Multiple thin-walled microcystic components (spongiform appearance) within >50% of the nodule [10, 11]
- Peripheral egg shell-type calcification [13]
- Isoechoic or slightly hyperechoic compared to the normal thyroid with peripheral hypoechoic halo [6]
- Peripheral vascularity or complete avascularity [11, 12]

4.3.1.2 Malignant Nodules
No individual feature is diagnostic but a combination of appearances aids in an accurate diagnosis of malignancy [7].

- Solid hypoechoic nodules with microcalcification (papillary thyroid cancer) [8].
- When imaged in transverse plane, the height is more than the width of the nodule (anterior posterior diameter > transverse diameter) [14, 15].
- Irregular margin, increased internal vascularity, and absence of halo [8].
- Follicular lesions more typically iso- or hyperechoic, homogenous with thick irregular halo [6, 8], and may not have microcalcification [16].
- Anaplastic cancers are usually large necrotic lesions with extrathyroidal extension [17].

4.4 Ultrasound Pitfalls

- The presence of multiple nodules should never be considered as a feature of benign disease. The risk of cancer is similar in multiple and solitary nodules [3]. In a study of 68 cases, 48% of malignancy was in multinodular goitres [18].
- Never dismiss small nodules.
- Lymph node metastases may have a different ultrasound appearance to the primary tumour. One study showed that 70% of papillary cancers lymph node metastases have a cystic component with a solid primary tumour [7].
- Don't misinterpret abnormal nodes adjacent to the thyroid gland as nodules in a multinodular goitre.
- Diffuse infiltrative malignancy may have similar appearances as autoimmune thyroiditis [7].

4.5 Mixed Solid Cystic Lesions

While cystic change is commonly seen in benign lesions, there is a small risk of cancer in mixed cystic solid lesions, and it is important to assess the solid component of the lesion. The lesion is more likely to be malignant if the total lesion is irregular and the solid component has microcalcification, non-central location, is hypoechoic and has taller than wider morphology [6].

4.6 FNAC of Thyroid Lesions

Various criteria have been published to aid in the diagnosis of thyroid cancer. For example, Kim et al. [19] criteria, the American Society of Clinical Endocrinologists Medical Guidelines [20] and the American Society of Radiologists in Ultrasound [21]. These criteria aim to guide in the decision-making as to which lesions require FNAC. The British Thyroid Society recommends an ultrasound (U) classification system to determine if a lesion should undergo FNAC. This is a U1–U5 grading system which helps distinguish benign from potentially malignant nodules [6].

Size is not a good criterion in determining if a lesion is malignant, and lesion morphology is considered much more useful in selection for FNAC [22, 23]. The patient's clinical history, risk factors, referring clinicians' opinion and multidisciplinary team (MDT) decision should influence the need for cytological assessment of a lesion.

Based on the ultrasound (U) criteria published by the British Thyroid Society, if a nodule is indeterminate, suspicious or malignant, it requires FNAC. Benign-appearing nodules do not need to be cytologically evaluated unless there is high clinical concern including high risk of malignancy.

If there is a suspicion of malignancy, then thorough examination of the neck should be performed, and any suspicious lymph nodes require FNAC.

4.7　Staging

Imaging plays an important role in the staging of thyroid cancer. Currently the most accepted system is the 6th edition of the American Joint Committee on Cancer (AJCC)/Union for International Cancer Control (UICC) classification which takes into consideration the TNM staging system and is based upon patient's age (varying depending on cut-off of 45 years) for papillary and follicular cancers. The medullary cancer staging is independent of age and is the same as that for the papillary and follicular cancer over 45 age group. Anaplastic cancers are all classified as stage 4 [5].

4.8　Primary Tumour Staging

According to the AJCC/UICC staging, ultrasound is the main imaging technique for stage T1 and T2 tumours. However, there is controversy in the case of multifocal disease as these deposits are very small and cannot all undergo FNAC. In this scenario, usually patients undergo total thyroidectomy.

MRI or CT is required for T3 and T4 stages as they assess extrathyroidal extension. MRI is preferred to CT, to avoid iodinated contrast as patients with differentiated tumours will require iodine 131 therapy post-surgery for residual disease or metastases. Patients with poorly differentiated tumours have no contraindication to iodinated contrast as they do not receive radioiodine therapy [5]. Imaging the primary cancer determines the treatment including if a tumour is resectable or irresectable and, if so, guides the surgeon to the extent of extrathyroidal spread and to which major structures may be involved. If >270° of the carotid artery or mediastinal vessels are involved, then the tumour is more likely to be unresectable [24].

4.9　Nodal Staging

Nodal staging is vital when planning surgery as there is good evidence that nodal metastases increase risk of local recurrence, and selective neck dissection should be performed [25, 26] . Ultrasound is the main imaging technique, and features of malignancy are rounded shape, loss of the hilum and peripheral vascularity. Nodal metastases are more common with papillary cancer, and in this case, they may show calcification, frequently small cystic change (20%) and hyperechogenicity (87%) [27, 28]. CT and MRI are potentially useful in the assessment of mediastinal nodes in patients with primary tumours invading with mediastinum, as well as patients with extensive central compartment nodes (level VI) nodes or lower cervical nodes on ultrasound [29].

4.10 Distant Metastases

Imaging for metastatic spread is performed postoperatively for differentiated cancers and preoperatively for anaplastic cancers. High-dose ablative iodine 131 therapy post-thyroidectomy not only ablates the remnant thyroid tissue but also detects nodal and metastatic disease at the same time as ablating any tumour foci. It should be noted that in some poorly differentiated papillary and follicular cancers, medullary and anaplastic tumours are iodine negative [5].

Follicular (which has propensity for haematological spread) and papillary cancers mainly metastasise to the lung and bone. Medullary cancer also metastasises to the liver surface which can be difficult to diagnose on imaging. Forty percent of anaplastic malignancies are metastatic at presentation.

CT chest will identify micronodular or macronodular pulmonary metastases. Some metastases are iodine negative although some iodine-positive foci are not visualised on CT [30]. Imaging with CT is usually performed in the postoperative period in patients with a persistently high thyroglobulin, negative 131/123 iodine scan, and in those with raised calcitonin in medullary cancer. CT also assesses for mediastinal nodes, bone lesions and liver metastases.

The role of FDG PET/CT is discussed elsewhere in the book. Other imaging modalities such as MRI, plain radiographs, ultrasound and bone scan may be useful for specific clinical scenarios. ^{111}In octreotide, Gallium 68 peptide imaging [31] and ^{131}I MIBG [32] have a role to play in medullary cancer particularly if targeted therapy is being considered.

Apart from radioiodine therapy, external beam including intensity-modulated radiotherapy is used to treat residual micro- or macroscopic disease. Imaging with CT and MRI is used for radiotherapy planning [33]

Approximately 25% of medullary cancers are familial, and imaging patients with the familial type should be screened for multiple endocrine neoplasia (MEN—type 11A commoner than 11B). Therefore, imaging has a role to play if parathyroid hyperplasia or pheochromocytoma is suspected [34].

4.11 Surveillance

^{131}I radioiodine ablative therapy is a standard post-surgery, and if the thyroglobulin levels (with thyroid-stimulating hormone stimulation) are undetectable and neck ultrasound postoperatively is normal, then further $^{131/123}$I scans are not required.

Ultrasound can detect disease which is iodine negative, and therefore yearly surveillance with cervical ultrasound even if thyroglobulin and calcitonin levels are undetectable [35] is advised.

If recurrence is suspected, then restaging is required usually with 123/131, ultrasound and CT/MRI. Potential problem is that the metastatic lymph nodes in papillary cancer can remain unchanged for years and also ablated nodes may also remain unchanged [5]. Additionally iodine scans have a limited role in less differentiated cancers, medullary and anaplastic cancers; hence, there is an increasing utilisation of FDG [36] and non-FDG PET/CT [37].

Key Points

- Thyroid lesions are commonly encountered in diagnostic radiology with reported incidence of 30–70% on ultrasound (less than 7% of thyroid nodules are malignant).

- The most important factor in managing a thyroid nodule is differentiating a benign lesion from a malignant nodule or identifying a malignant nodule in the setting of a multinodular goitre.

- Ultrasound is the most commonly used modality in the primary diagnosis and assessment of the thyroid.

- CT and MRI are inferior in the detection and characterisation of thyroid nodules, and the roles of these modalities are to assess for extrathyroidal tumour extension, nodal disease and distant metastases.

- Thyroid cancer may have variable imaging characteristics on ultrasound, and it may be difficult to differentiate from a benign nodule.

- The presence of multiple nodules should never be considered as a feature of benign disease.

- Cystic change is commonly seen in benign lesions, there is a small risk of cancer in mixed cystic solid lesions, and it is important to assess the solid component of the lesion.

- The lesion is more likely to be malignant if the total lesion is irregular and the solid component has microcalcification and non-central location, is hypoechoic and has taller than wider morphology.

- Size is not a good criterion in determining if a lesion is malignant, and lesion morphology is considered much more useful in selection for FNAC.

- The patient's clinical history, risk factors, referring clinician's opinion and multidisciplinary team (MDT) decision should influence the need for cytological assessment of a lesion.

- According to the AJCC/UICC staging, ultrasound is the main imaging technique for stage T1 and T2 tumours.

- MRI or CT is required for T3 and T4 stages as they assess extrathyroidal extension. MRI is preferred to CT, to avoid iodinated contrast as patients with differentiated tumours will require iodine 131 therapy post-surgery for residual disease or metastases.

- Patients with poorly differentiated tumours have no contraindication to iodinated contrast as they do not receive radioiodine therapy.

- Nodal staging is vital when planning surgery as there is good evidence that nodal metastases increase risk of local recurrence, and selective neck dissection should be performed.

- Ultrasound is the main imaging technique, and features of nodal malignancy are rounded shape, loss of the hilum and peripheral vascularity.

- Imaging for metastatic spread is performed postoperatively for differentiated cancers and preoperatively for anaplastic cancers.

- CT chest will identify micronodular or macronodular pulmonary metastases. Some metastases are iodine negative although some iodine-positive foci are not visualised on CT.

- Imaging with CT is usually performed in the postoperative period in patients with a persistently high thyroglobulin, negative 131/123 iodine scan and in those with raised calcitonin in medullary cancer.

References

1. Davies L, Welch HG. Increasing incidence of thyroid cancer in the United States, 1973-2002. 2006;295(18):2164-2167.
2. Frates MC, Benson CB, Charbonneau JW. Management of thyroid nodules detected at US: society of radiologists in ultrasound consensus statement. Radiology. 2005;237:794–800.
3. Papini E, Guglielmi R, Bianchini A, et al. Risk of malignancy in nonpalpable thyroid nodules: predictive value of ultrasound and color-Doppler features. J Clin Endocrinol Metab. 2002;87(5):1941–6.
4. Hambly NM, Gonen M, Gerst SR. Implementation of Evidence-based guidelines for thyroid nodule biopsy: a model for establishment of practice standards. Am J Roentgenol. 2011;196:655–60.
5. King AD. Imaging for staging and management of thyroid cancer. Cancer Imaging. 2008;8(1):57–69.
6. Perros P, Boelaert K, Colley S, Evans C, Evans RM, Gerrard Ba G, Gilbert J, Harrison B, Johnson SJ, Giles TE, Moss L, Lewington V, Newbold K, Taylor J, Thakker RV, Watkinson J, Williams GR, British Thyroid Association. Management of thyroid cancer. Clin Endocrinol (Oxf). 2014;81(Suppl 1):1–122. https://doi.org/10.1111/cen.12515.

7. Hoang JK, Lee WK, Lee M, Johnson D, Farrell S. US features of thyroid malignancy: pearls and pitfalls. RSNA Educ Exhibits. 2007;27(3).
8. American Thyroid Association (ATA) Guidelines Taskforce on Thyroid Nodules and Differentiated Thyroid Cancer, Cooper DS, Doherty GM, Haugen BR, Kloos RT, Lee SL, Mandel SJ, Mazzaferri EL, McIver B, Pacini F, Schlumberger M, Sherman SI, Steward DL, Tuttle RM. Revised American Thyroid Association management guidelines for patients with thyroid nodules and differentiated thyroid cancer. Thyroid. 2009 Nov;19(11):1167–214.
9. Frates MC, Benson CB, Doubilet PM, Kunreuther E, Contreras M, Cibas ES, Orcutt J, Moore FD Jr, Larsen PR, Marqusee E, Alexander EK. Prevalence and distribution of carcinoma in patients with solitary and multiple thyroid nodules on sonography. J Clin Endocrinol Metab. 2006;91:3411–7.
10. Bonavita JA, Mayo J, Babb J, Bennett G, Oweity T, Macari M, Yee J. Pattern recognition of benign nodules at ultrasound of the thyroid: which nodules can be left alone? AJR Am J Roentgenol. 2009;193:207–13.
11. Moon WJ, Jung SL, Lee JH, Na DG, Baek JH, Lee YH, Kim J, Kim HS, Byun JS, Lee DH, Thyroid Study Group, Korean Society of Neuro-and Head and Neck Radiology. Benign and malignant thyroid nodules: US differentiation—multicenter retrospective study. Radiology. 2008;247:762–70.
12. Chan BK, Desser TS, IR MD, Weigel RJ, Jeffrey RB Jr. Common and uncommon sonographic features of papillary thyroid carcinoma. J Ultrasound Med. 2003;22(10):1083–10913.
13. Kim BK, Choi YS, Kwon HJ, et al. Relationships between patterns of calcification in thyroid nodules and histopathologic findings. Endocr J. 2013;60:155–60.
14. Leenhardt L, Hejblum G, Franc B, Fediaevsky LD, Delbot T, Le Guillouzic D, Ménégaux F, Guillausseau C, Hoang C, Turpin G, Aurengo A. Indications and limits of ultrasound-guided cytology in the management of nonpalpable thyroid nodules. J Clin Endocrinol Metab. 1999;84:24–8.
15. Ahn SS, Kim E-K, Kang DR. Biopsy of thyroid nodules: comparison of three sets of guidelines. Am J Roentgenol. 2010;194:31–7.
16. Moon WJ, Kwag HJ, Na DG. Are there any specific ultrasound findings of nodular hyperplasia ("leave me alone" lesion) to differentiate it from follicular adenoma? Acta Radiol. 2009;50:383–8.
17. Kebebew E, Greenspan FS, Clark OH, Woeber KA, McMillan A. Anaplastic thyroid carcinoma. Treatment outcome and prognostic factors. Cancer. 2005;103:1330–5.
18. Jun P, Chow LC, Jeffrey RB. The sonographic features of papillary thyroid carcinomas: pictorial essay. Ultrasound Q. 2005;21(1):39–45.
19. Kim EK, Park CS, Chung WY, et al. New sonographic criteria for recommending fine-needle aspiration biopsy of nonpalpable solid nodules of the thyroid. Am J Roentgenol. 2002;178:687–91.
20. Gharib H, Papini E, Duick D, et al. American association of clinical endocrinologist, associatione medici endocrinologi, and European thyroid association, medical guidelines for clinical practice for the diagnosis and management of thyroid nodules. Endocr Pract. 2006;12(1):63–102.
21. Frates MC, Benson CB, Charboneau JW, Cibas ES. Management of thyroid nodules detected at US: Society of Radiologists in Ultrasound consensus conference statement. Radiology. 2005;237(3):794–800.
22. Choi SH, Han KH, Yoon JH, et al. Factors affecting inadequate sampling of ultrasound-guided fine-needle aspiration biopsy of thyroid nodules. Clin Endocrinol (Oxf). 2011;74:776–782.23.
23. Aron M, Mallik A, Verma K. Fine needle aspiration cytology of follicular variant of papillary carcinoma of the thyroid: morphologic pointers to its diagnosis. Acta Cytol. 2006;50:663–8.
24. Yousem DM, Hatabu H, Hurst RW, et al. Carotid artery invasion by head and neck masses: prediction with MR imaging. Radiology. 1995;195:715–20.
25. Noguchi S, Murakami N, Yamashita H, Toda M, Kawamoto H. Papillary thyroid carcinoma: modified radical neck dissection improves prognosis. Arch Surg. 1998;133:276–80.
26. Palazzo FF, Gosnell J, Savio R, et al. Lymphadenectomy for papillary thyroid cancer: changes in practice over four decades. Eur J Surg Oncol. 2006;32:340–4.

27. Ahuja AT, Chow L, Chik W, King W, Metreweli C. Metastatic cervical nodes in papillary carcinoma of the thyroid: ultrasound and histological correlation. Clin Radiol. 1995;50:229–31.
28. Rosario PW, de Faria S, Bicalho L, et al. Ultrasonographic differentiation between metastatic and benign lymph nodes in patients with papillary thyroid carcinoma. J Ultrasound Med. 2005;24:1385–9.
29. Sugenoya A, Asanuma K, Shingu K, et al. Clinical evaluation of upper mediastinal dissection for differentiated thyroid carcinoma. Surgery. 1993;113:541–5.
30. Küçük ON, Gültekin SS, Aras G, Ibiş E. Radioiodine whole-body scans, thyroglobulin levels, 99mTc-MIBI scans and computed tomography: results in patients with lung metastases from differentiated thyroid cancer. Nucl Med Commun. 2006;27(3):261–6.
31. Conry BG, Papathanasiou ND, Prakash V, et al. Comparison of (68)Ga-DOTATATE and (18) F-fluorodeoxyglucose PET/CT in the detection of recurrent medullary thyroid carcinoma. Eur J Nucl Med Mol Imaging. 2010;37(1):49–57.
32. Castellani MR, Seregni E, Maccauro M. etal MIBG for diagnosis and therapy of medullary thyroid carcinoma: is there still a role? J. Nucl Med Mol Imaging. 2008;52(4):430–40.
33. Int Rosenbluth BD, Serrano V, Happersett L, et al. Intensity-modulated radiation therapy for the treatment of nonanaplastic thyroid cancer. J Radiat Oncol Biol Phys. 2005;63(5):1419–26.
34. National Cancer Institute guidance. Thyroid cancer
35. Antonelli A, Miccoli P, Ferdeghini M, et al. Role of neck ultrasonography in the follow-up of patients operated on for thyroid cancer. Thyroid. 1995;5(1):25–8.
36. Ozkan E, Soydal C, Kucuk ON, Ibis E, Erbay G. Impact of ^{18}F-FDG PET/CT for detecting recurrence of medullary thyroid carcinoma. Nucl Med Commun. 2011;32(12):1162–8.
37. Marcus C, Whitworth PW, Surasi DS, Pai SI, Subramaniam RM. PET/CT in the management of thyroid cancer. AJR Am J Roentgenol. 2014;202(6):1316–29. https://doi.org/10.2214/AJR.13.11673.

Radionuclide Imaging in Thyroid Cancer

Emmanouil Panagiotidis

Contents

5.1	Introduction	35
5.2	Primary Diagnosis/Thyroid Scan	36
5.3	Thyroid Nodules	37
5.4	Scintigraphy for Staging/Restaging of Differentiated Thyroid Carcinoma	39
References		43

5.1 Introduction

Molecular imaging plays an important role not only in the diagnosis of thyroid cancer but also in the evaluation and clinical management. The transition from the previous routine use of the thyroid scan to its limited role nowadays has led to significant alteration of the contemporary nuclear medicine; the dosimetry in combination with the theranostic approach of the personalised medicine has led to new medical horizons. Although the SPECT tracers have been acknowledged as the mainstream for thyroid cancer therapy, the emergence of the new PET radiotracers, apart from the 18F-fluorodeoxyglucose (FDG), such as 11C-methionine, 68Ga-somatostatin receptor binding agents and more interestingly ^{124}I, which however is not still widely available yet, will bring broader applicability.

The use of radioactive iodine for both diagnostic and therapeutic purposes of thyroid cancer has been signalled by the birth of nuclear medicine as speciality in the 1940s and has been the standard treatment for differentiated thyroid cancer even

E. Panagiotidis
Department of Nuclear Medicine, Royal Liverpool University Hospital, Liverpool, UK
e-mail: mpanagiotidis@gmail.com

nowadays, despite the fact that numerous interventions have been considered as replacements for radioactive iodine therapy, without success. Moreover, although the routine use of thyroid scans in all thyroid nodules is no longer recommended, in the initial workup of a thyroid nodule, radioiodine imaging can be particularly helpful especially when the thyroid-stimulating hormone level is low and an autonomously functioning nodule is suspected or in case needle aspiration biopsy is indeterminate.

5.2 Primary Diagnosis/Thyroid Scan

Despite the fact that thyroid cancer is uncommon malignancy, thyroid nodules are very common and pose an often clinical dilemma with a prevalence of palpable thyroid nodules in 4–7% of various populations [1–4].However, only 1 out of 20 clinically identified nodules is malignant with the prevalence of predominately nonpalpable thyroid nodules as depicted by ultrasonography (US) being very high as many as 50–70% [5–7]. The incidence of thyroid cancer continues to rise, with a 2.4-fold increase in incidence since 1975, based largely upon detection of small ($\leq$2 cm) tumours, which represent 87% of newly diagnosed cases [8].

It is well established that clinical examination and serum TSH assessment in combination with US are the appropriate primary evaluation processes, while fine needle aspiration cytology (FNAC) is the most reliable technique for the diagnosis of thyroid nodule or nodular goitre [9]. Adding data obtained from the use of scintigraphy with technetium-99m pertechnetate (99mTcO4) could help in establishing a diagnosis since a hyperfunctioning nodule is extremely rare and malignant and a hypofunctioning nodule with features of a small cyst on USS and benign features on FNA could be reassuringly monitored, while a large and complex cyst or a multinodular goitre with a dominant nodule may raise suspicion of malignancy. The common indications for thyroid scan are mentioned in Table 5.1 [10].

The most common and practical method for thyroid scintigraphy is gamma camera planar imaging using 99mTcO4 as a radiotracer. The uptake mechanism is due to trapping of 3–4% of the administered activity, usually 80 MBq which results in good-quality images, without the tracer to undergo further metabolic degradation in the thyroid cells, in contrast to iodine, which is both trapped and organified by follicular cells, which mimics more the physiological approach (Table 5.1.1). However both iodine tracers ^{131}I and ^{123}I have logistic and practical issues that interfere to the daily clinical practice, being both of them superseded by 99mTcO4, either for high

Table 5.1 Common indications for thyroid scan

1. Assessment of functionality of thyroid nodules
2. Assessment of goitre including hyperthyroid goitre
3. Assessment of uptake function prior to radioiodine treatment
4. Assessment of ectopic thyroid tissue
5. Assessment of suspected thyroiditis
6. Assessment of neonatal hypothyroidism

radiation burden and noisy images for the ^{131}I or for availability for ^{123}I as a cyclotron product.

The use of ^{123}I and ^{131}I for thyroid imaging permits evaluation of the entire metabolic iodine pathway including trapping, organification, coupling, hormone storage and secretion [11]. Both ^{123}I and 99mTcO4 are trapped by follicular thyroid cells, salivary glands, choroid plexus, gastric parietal cells and lactating mammary glands. Recognition of these sites is important, especially when thyroid ectopic tissue is suspected. The commonly depicted uniform 'butterfly'-shaped thyroid is not always visualised, as variations in size and shape of both lobes are not uncommon.

^{123}I is the agent of choice when evaluating substernal goitres because there is usually substantial mediastinal blood pool activity associated with 99mTcO4. The uptake of radioiodine by the follicular trapping system is decreased by perchlorate, thiocyanate ions and expansion of the circulating iodine pool from dietary and medical sources (IV contrast, amiodarone) [12].

Other radiopharmaceuticals, with different mechanisms of uptake, include 201Tl or 99mTc-MIBI which is used in the assessment of hypofunctioning nodules and postsurgical follow-up especially in non-iodine-avid thyroid carcinoma (Table 5.2).

5.3 Thyroid Nodules

Based upon their scintigraphic appearance, nodules can be classified as hypofunctioning, hyperfunctioning or functioning. A hypofunctioning nodule demonstrates decreased tracer uptake compared to the surrounding normal thyroid tissue [11]. A hypofunctioning nodule reflects lack of organification (or trapping if Tc-pertechnetate is the imaging agent) and subsequent thyroxine synthesis. The great majority of solitary thyroid nodules are hypofunctioning, but only 10–25% of these are malignant [12]. Thyroid cancers appear as hypofunctioning nodules due to altered iodine metabolism characterised by decreased iodine uptake and markedly reduced iodine organification [13] (Tables 5.3 and 5.4).

A hyperfunctioning nodule has greater activity than the normal surrounding thyroid tissue. Differential diagnoses for the hyperfunctioning nodules include benign hyperfunctioning follicular adenomas, adenomatous hyperplasia, compensatory hypertrophy and physiologic thyroid hyperplasia. The probability of cancer in a hyperfunctioning nodule scanned with radioiodine is less than 4% [14].

There is a possibility for a nodule to be hyperfunctioning on 99mTcO4 but hypofunctioning on ^{123}I study, known as discordant nodule. The discordant nodules' mechanism could be explained by either the Tc-pertechnetate trapping preservation in combination with failure of organification or the rapid release of organified iodine from the nodule [15]. Solitary discordant thyroid nodules are generally considered to be rare (2–8%), and cases of discrepancy between the 99mTcO4 and ^{123}I studies appear most often in multinodular goitres [15, 16]. Although early studies showed that as many as 30% of discordant nodules may be malignant, discrepancies are also far more likely to be caused by benign thyroid disorders rather than malignancy [15, 17]. The pitfalls in thyroid scan reporting are mentioned in Table 5.5.

Table 5.2 Characteristics of radiopharmaceuticals used for thyroid scintigraphy

Radiopharmaceutical	Half-life (hours)	Energy (KeV)	Administered dose (MBq)	Trapping	Organification	Cost	Availability	Dietary restriction	Quality Image
99mTcO4	6	140	80	Yes only	No	Low	Easy	No	Good
131I	192	364	37	Yes	Yes	Low	Limited	Yes	Noisy
123I	13	159	185	Yes	Yes	High	Limited	Yes	Good

Table 5.3 Differential considerations of a hypofunctioning nodule [11]

Benign (80%)
Simple cyst
Adenomatous hyperplasia
Focal haemorrhage
Inflammatory
Focal thyroiditis
Abscess
Parathyroid adenoma
Malignant (20%)
Thyroid carcinoma
Parathyroid adenoma/carcinoma
Thyroid lymphoma
Metastatic disease

Table 5.4 Factors increasing the malignancy risk in hypofunctioning nodule [18]

1. History of radiotherapy to the head and neck
2. Lymphadenopathy in the neck
3. Age: less than 20 years (about twofold increased risk) or over 60 years (about sixfold increased risk)
4. Male sex: two times greater than females
5. Evidence of local invasion: recurrent laryngeal nerve involvement – voice hoarseness
6. Size of nodule: greater than 4 cm
7. Nodule enlarges, especially while on thyroxine suppression: most benign nodules will decrease in size or remain unchanged
8. Family history of thyroid cancer
9. MEN 2 syndrome

Table 5.5 Pitfalls in reporting thyroid scans

1. Activity in the oesophagus
2. Failure to correlate the finding of clinical palpation and ultrasound examination with the radionuclide scan
3. Low or absent uptake due to block by
   - Iingested or administered iodine
   - Iodine containing medication
   - Thyroxine (levothyroxine sodium) medication

The size of nodules that can be detected by pertechnetate imaging depends upon the nodule function and size. Hyperfunctioning nodules may be seen even if they are very small, but a hypofunctioning nodule less than 0.8–1.0 cm in size lying within the gland may not be discernible [1]. In general, pertechnetate 5-mm pinhole imaging has a sensitivity of 80–95% for hypofunctioning nodules between 8 and 18 mm but nearly 0% for nodules less than 5 mm.

5.4 Scintigraphy for Staging/Restaging of Differentiated Thyroid Carcinoma

In patients being considered for ablation therapy, a pretreatment. low-dose ^{131}I (111–185 MBq/3–5 mCi) diagnostic whole-body scintigraphy (dxWBS) can be performed 5–6 weeks following surgery to assess for the presence of metastatic lesions. Either thyroid hormone withdrawal or thyrogen stimulation (human recombinant TSH) can be used for patient preparation for the initial diagnostic scan, as long as there is no evidence of metastatic disease, aiming for TSH levels more than 30 IU/mL [19]. If the radioiodine uptake of the neck region is above 15% revealing a significant amount of thyroid remnant tissue, then a revision or completion thyroidectomy should be considered. However a dxWBS is not always necessary, especially in cases which the total thyroidectomy has been performed by an experienced surgeon in low-risk patients who have no clinical evidence of tumour after surgery [13, 20].

The sensitivity and specificity for the detection of thyroid cancer recurrences or metastases of planar dxWBS ^{131}I imaging range between 45 and 75% and 96 and 100%, respectively (depending on the activity dose administered) [21–26]. However, due to the lack of anatomic landmarks and low count statistics, the precise localisation of the radioactive foci can be difficult to be ascertained on planar images [27], despite the fact that SPECT images provide better contrast resolution.

SPECT/CT is a powerful diagnostic tool which allows precise localisation of radioactivity and improved characterisation of benign and malignant radioactivity distributions compared to planar imaging. In conjunction with pre-ablation or post-therapy dxWBS, SPECT/CT has been used for completion of thyroid cancer staging. The impact on clinical management is important providing prognostic information by detecting a greater number of lesions than planar imaging such as lymph node metastases adjacent to residual thyroid tissue or the salivary glands and by increasing reader confidence in the identification of physiologic foci of tracer uptake and therefore improving specificity with decreased false-positive findings and in improved localisation of metastatic sites [21, 27–30].

Several studies have shown the high impact of the SPECT/CT imaging in altering clinical management in 57–74% of patients especially in selection of ^{131}I dose and in guiding surgical management, particularly in differentiating thyroid bed activity from adjacent lymph nodes [21, 27, 29].

Disadvantages of SPECT/CT include additional imaging time, possible patient discomfort and claustrophobia from lying in a confined position for approximately 20 min in the tightly enclosed space of the SPECT/CT gantry, low spatial resolution of SPECT limited by the partial volume effect in small lesions and the fact that evaluation of both neck and distant radioactive foci may require two separate SPECT/CT acquisitions and additional radiation exposure from the CT component of the study (1–4 mSv with each acquisition) [31].

Some limitations of SPECT/CT are related to the low intrinsic activity of ^{131}I scans that can produce very low count images, and this can result in image misregistration [27].

False-negative scans (up to 22% of patients) can occur in patients due to small lesion size and in non-iodine-avid disease (20–30% of patients) such as Hurthle cell thyroid cancer, papillary thyroid cancer with unfavourable histology (tall cell, columnar or cribriform variants) or poorly differentiated thyroid cancer (such as trabecular, insular or solid variants) [29].

False-positive scans can occur in patients due to local contamination (clothing, skin, hair, collimator, imaging table), oesophageal activity, asymmetric salivary gland activity, breast uptake, thymus uptake, renal activity and bowel activity [29].

Another radioiodine isotope, iodine-123 (^{123}I), may also be used for diagnostic imaging (1.5–3 mCi), with the advantages of a lower-energy gamma emission and less likelihood for thyroidal tissue stunning, a phenomenon whereby a diagnostic dose of radioiodine decreases the uptake of a subsequent therapeutic dose by remnant thyroid tissue or by functioning metastatic deposits. Using low-energy (159 KeV), high-resolution collimators permits acquisition of high-quality images. Drawbacks to the use of ^{123}I are higher costs and a short half-life of 13 h, precluding multiday imaging and increasing the complexity of the dosimetry calculation.

According to the American Thyroid Association, imaging before ^{131}I therapy is not recommended, unless the extent of the thyroid remnant cannot be accurately ascertained from the surgical report or neck ultrasonography or when the results would alter either the decision to treat or the activity of RAI that is administered [32]. However there are few but definite clinical issues that pretherapy scanning can uncover such as occult metastases, large thyroid remnants and distant metastases in the brain or spinal cord that necessitate pre-radiation corticosteroid administration that leads either to ^{131}I dose titration or clinical management alteration, for example, external beam radiotherapy (EBRT) or second surgical intervention.

The post-^{131}I ablation scintigraphy is recommended 4–10 days post-therapy administration, providing enhanced sensitivity over all the pre-ablative imaging methods, due to high dosage in conjunction with SPECT/CT improving tumour localisation.

Key Points

- Molecular imaging plays an important role not only in the diagnosis of thyroid cancer but also in the evaluation and clinical management.
- The most common and practical method for thyroid scintigraphy is gamma camera planar imaging using 99mTcO4 as a radiotracer.
- The use of ^{123}I and ^{131}I for thyroid imaging permits evaluation of the entire metabolic iodine pathway including trapping, organification, coupling, hormone storage and secretion.
- Based upon their scintigraphic appearance, nodules can be classified as hypofunctioning, hyperfunctioning or functioning.
- The great majority of solitary thyroid nodules are hypofunctioning, but only 10–25% of these are malignant.

- The probability of cancer in a hyperfunctioning nodule scanned with radioiodine is less than 4%.

- The size of nodules that can be detected by pertechnetate imaging depends upon the nodules function and size, and hypofunctioning nodule less than 0.8–1.0 cm in size lying within the gland may not be discernible.

- In patients being considered for ablation therapy, a pretreatment. low-dose ^{131}I (111–185 MBq/3–5 mCi) diagnostic whole-body scintigraphy (dxWBS) can be performed 5–6 weeks following surgery to assess for the presence of metastatic lesions.

- The sensitivity and specificity for the detection of thyroid cancer recurrences or metastases of planar dxWBS ^{131}I imaging range between 45 and 75% and 96 and 100%, respectively (depending on the activity dose administered).

- SPECT/CT is a powerful diagnostic tool which allows precise localisation of radioactivity and improved characterisation of benign and malignant radioactivity distributions compared to planar imaging.

- Several studies have shown the high impact of the SPECT/CT imaging in altering clinical management in 57–74% of patients especially in selection of ^{131}I dose and in guiding surgical management, particularly in differentiating thyroid bed activity from adjacent lymph nodes.

- False-negative scans (up to 22% of patients) can occur in patients due to small lesion size and in non-iodine-avid disease (20–30% of patients) such as Hurthle cell thyroid cancer, papillary thyroid cancer with unfavourable histology (tall cell, columnar or cribriform variants) or poorly differentiated thyroid cancer (such as trabecular, insular or solid variants).

- False-positive scans can occur in patients due to local contamination (clothing, skin, hair, collimator, imaging table), oesophageal activity, asymmetric salivary gland activity, breast uptake, thymus uptake, renal activity and bowel activity.

- According to the American Thyroid Association, imaging before ^{131}I therapy is not recommended, unless the extent of the thyroid remnant cannot be accurately ascertained from the surgical report or neck ultrasonography or when the results would alter either the decision to treat or the activity of RAI that is administered

- Post-131I ablation scintigraphy is recommended 4–10 days post-therapy administration.

References

1. Cappelli C, Castellano M, Pirola I, Gandossi E, De Martino E, Cumetti D, et al. Thyroid nodule shape suggests malignancy. Eur J Endocrinol. 2006;155:27–31.
2. Ezzal S, Sarti DA, Cain DR, Braunstein GD. Thyroid incidentalomas: Prevalence by palpation and ultrasonography. Arch Intern Med. 1994;154:1338–40.
3. Brander A, Viikinkoski P, Nickels J, Kivisaari L. Thyroid gland: US screening in a random adult population. Radiology. 1995;181:683–7.
4. Wienke JR, Chong WK, Fielding JR, Zou KH, Mittelstaedt CA. Sonographic features of benign thyroid nodules. J Ultrasound Med. 2003;22:1027–31.
5. Hay ID, Grant CS, Van Heerden JA, Goellner JR, Ebersold JR, Bergstralh EJ. Papillary thyroid microcarcinoma: a study of 535 cases observed in a 50-year period. Surgery. 1994;112:1139–47.
6. Tourniaire J, Bernard MH, Bizzolon-Roblin MH, Bertholon-Gregoire M, Berger-Dutrieux N. 1998 Papillary microcarcinoma of the thyroid. 179 cases reported since. Presse Med. 1973;27:1467–9.
7. Papini E, Guglielmi R, Bianchini A, Crescenzi A, Taccagna S, Nardi F, et al. Risk of malignancy in nonpalpable thyroid nodules: Predictive value of ultrasound and color-doppler features. J Clin Endocrinol Metabol. 2002;87:1941–6.
8. Davies L, Welch HG. Increasing incidence of thyroid cancer in the United States, 1973–2002. JAMA. 2006;295(18):2164–7.
9. Cibas ES, Ali SZ. The Bethesda System for reporting thyroid cytopathology. Thyroid. 2009;19:1159–65.
10. Sarkar SD, Becker DV. Thyroid uptake and imaging. In: Becker KL, editor. Principles and practice of endocrinology and metabolism. Philadelphia: JB Lippincott; 1995. p. 307–13.
11. Shulkin BL, Shapiro B. The role of imaging tests in the diagnosis of thyroid carcinoma. Endocrinol Metab Clin North Am. 1990;19:523–41.
12. Charles MD. Thyroid and whole body imaging. In: Ingbar SH, Braverman LE, editors. The thyroid. 5th ed. Philadelphia: Lippincott; 1986. p. 458–78.
13. Robbins RJ, et al. The evolving role of 131I for the treatment of differentiated thyroid carcinoma. J Nucl Med. 2005;46:28S–37S.
14. Price DC. Radioisotopic evaluation of the thyroid and the parathyroids. Radiol Clin North Am. 1993;31:991–1015.
15. Kusic Z, et al. Comparison of technetium-99m and iodine-123 imaging of thyroid nodules: Correlation with pathologic findings. J Nucl Med. 1990;31:393–9.
16. Intenzo CM, et al. Scintigraphic manifestations of thyrotoxicosis. Radiographics. 2003;23:857–69.
17. Freitas JE, Freitas AE. Thyroid and parathyroid imaging. Semin Nucl Med. 1994;24:234–45.
18. Belfiore A, et al. Cancer risk in patients with cold thyroid nodules: Relevance of iodine intake, sex, age, and multinodularity. Am J Med. 1992;93:363–9.
19. Van Nostrand D, et al. Recombinant human thyroid-stimulating hormone versus thyroid hormone withdrawal in the identification of metastasis in differentiated thyroid cancer with 131I planar whole-body imaging and 124I PET. J Nucl Med. 2012;53:359–62.
20. Mazzaferri EL. Empirically treating high serum thyroglobulin levels. J Nucl Med. 2005;46:1079–88.
21. Spanu A, et al. 131I SPECT/CT in the follow-up of differentiated thyroid carcinoma: incremental value versus planar imaging. J Nucl Med. 2009;50:184–90.
22. Tharp K, Israel O, Hausmann J, Bettman L, Martin WH, Daitzchman M, et al. Impact of 131I-SPECT/CT images obtained with an integrated system in the follow-up of patients with thyroid carcinoma. Eur J Nucl Med Mol Imaging. 2004;31(10):1435–42.
23. Delbeke D, Schoder H, Martin WH, Wahl RL. Hybrid imaging (SPECT/CT and PET/CT): improving therapeutic decisions. Semin Nucl Med. 2009;39(5):308–40.

24. Filesi M, Signore A, Ventroni G, Melacrinis FF, Ronga G. Role of initial iodine-131 whole-body scan and serum thyroglobulin in differentiated thyroid carcinoma metastases. J Nucl Med. 1998;39(9):1542–6.
25. Lind P, Kohlfurst S. Respective roles of thyroglobulin, radioiodine imaging, and positron emission tomography in the assessment of thyroid cancer. Semin Nucl Med. 2006;36(3):194–205.
26. Van Sorge-van Boxtel RA, van Eck-Smit BL, Goslings BM. Comparison of serum thyroglobulin, 131I and 201Tl scintigraphy in the postoperative follow-up of differentiated thyroid cancer. Nucl Med Commun. 1993;14(5):365–72.
27. Wong KK, et al. Staging of differentiated thyroid carcinoma using diagnostic 131I SPECT/CT. AJR Am J Roentgenol. 2010;195:730–6.
28. Schmidt D, et al. Impact of 131I SPECT/spiral CT on nodal staging of differentiated thyroid carcinoma at the first radioablation. J Nucl Med. 2009;50:18–23.
29. Avram AM. Radioiodine scintigraphy with SPECT/CT: an important diagnostic tool for thyroid cancer staging and risk stratification. J Nucl Med. 2012;53:754–64.
30. Maruoka Y, et al. Incremental diagnostic value of SPECT/CT with 131I scintigraphy after radioiodine therapy in patients with well-differentiated thyroid carcinoma. Radiology. 2012;265:902–9.
31. Buck AK, Nekolla SG, Ziegler SI, Drzezga A. SPECT/CT. J Nucl Med. 2008;49(8):1305–19.
32. American Thyroid Association (ATA) Guidelines Taskforce on Thyroid Nodules, Cooper DS, Doherty GM, Haugen BR, Kloos RT, Lee SL, Mandel SJ, Mazzaferri EL, McIver B, Pacini F, Schlumberger M, Sherman SI, Steward DL, Tuttle RM. Revised American Thyroid Association management guidelines for patients with thyroid nodules and differentiated thyroid cancer. Thyroid. 2009 Nov;19(11):1167–214.

18F-FDG PET/CT Normal Variants, Artefacts and Pitfalls in Thyroid Cancer

Arun Sasikumar, Alexis Corrigan, Muhammad Umar Khan, and Gopinath Gnanasegaran

Contents

6.1	Introduction	45
6.2	Head and Neck	46
	6.2.1 Technical: Artefacts and Pitfalls	46
	6.2.2 Thyroid: Variants, Artefacts and Pitfalls	46
	6.2.3 Head and Neck: Variants, Artefacts and Pitfalls	49
References		59

6.1 Introduction

18F-FDG is widely used as a PET tracer in UK oncologic clinical practice. 18F-FDG has the potential to be a specific and sensitive test with clear indications in the management of thyroid malignancy [1]. PET/CT is a whole body technique, and the normal distribution, common artefact, variant and pitfalls of 18F-FDG PET/CT have been extensively described [2–4]. In this chapter we will give an overview of the more commonly seen variants and artefacts, particularly within the context of assessment of thyroid malignancy.

A. Sasıkumar (✉)
Consultant and Head of the Department, Department of Nuclear Medicine,
St Gregorios International Cancer Care Centre, Parumala, Kerala, India
e-mail: sasikumararun@gmail.com

A. Corrigan
Consultant in Radionuclide Radiology, Maidstone Hospital, Maidstone, UK

M.U. Khan
Al-Jahra Hospital, Al-Jahra, Kuwait

G. Gnanasegaran
Department of Nuclear Medicine, Royal Free London NHS Foundation Trust, London, UK

© Springer International Publishing AG, part of Springer Nature 2018
S. Vinjamuri (ed.), *PET/CT in Thyroid Cancer*, Clinicians' Guides to Radionuclide Hybrid Imaging, https://doi.org/10.1007/978-3-319-71846-0_6

The biodistribution of FDG can vary according to fasting state, level of muscular exertion, various medications and the length of the uptake period after injection [5]. Rigorous attention should be given to the preparation of patients prior to ^{18}F-FDG PET/CT [6, 7]. Diabetic patients in particular require careful preparation.

^{18}F-FDG accumulation is not specific to cancer cells, and awareness of normal biodistribution, variants and common benign pathology that may mimic malignancy is required for accurate interpretation of PET/CT examinations.

Activated inflammatory processes also show increased glycolysis and consequently FDG uptake [5, 8].

6.2 Head and Neck

6.2.1 Technical: Artefacts and Pitfalls

In the assessment of thyroid and other head and neck malignancies, the major technical challenge is limiting voluntary patient movement in the head and neck region. Motion artefacts commonly arise from either motion of the head during the PET acquisition or from movement that occurs between the two acquisitions. Motion during the CT acquisition is less common as the CT acquisition is relatively quick. It is usual in many centres to perform PET imaging in the assessment of head and neck malignancy with a specific head restraint to improve patient comfort and compliance, which also helps to limit motion. If local movement is severe, repeat local imaging may be required (Table 6.1).

Local CT artefacts from dental implants or fillings can cause difficulties both related to localisation and beam hardening artefact, resulting in inappropriate attenuation correction (Fig. 6.1). Review of other imaging modalities and the non-attenuation correction imaging, respectively, can mitigate these problems.

6.2.2 Thyroid: Variants, Artefacts and Pitfalls

The incidence of thyroid malignancy is related to a variety of risk factors. In general age and sex are common risk factors for a variety of cancer types. When analysing studies, particularly for older patients, the reporter must also be alert to the potential for detection of additional incidental malignancy.

Table 6.1 Common technical problems affecting ^{18}F-FDG PET/CT in the head and neck region

	Appearance	Reason	Comment
Voluntary motion	Blurred PET image	PET image represents average of all motion	Communication, support and restraints. Repeat local view
Recent intervention (biopsy or surgery)	Locally increased or decreased uptake	Inflammatory reaction, haematoma, seroma	Delay PET imaging, if possible. Correlate with medical record
Artefact from metalwork or dental amalgam	Locally increased or decreased uptake	AC error due to CT metal artefact	Review non-attenuation corrected imaging

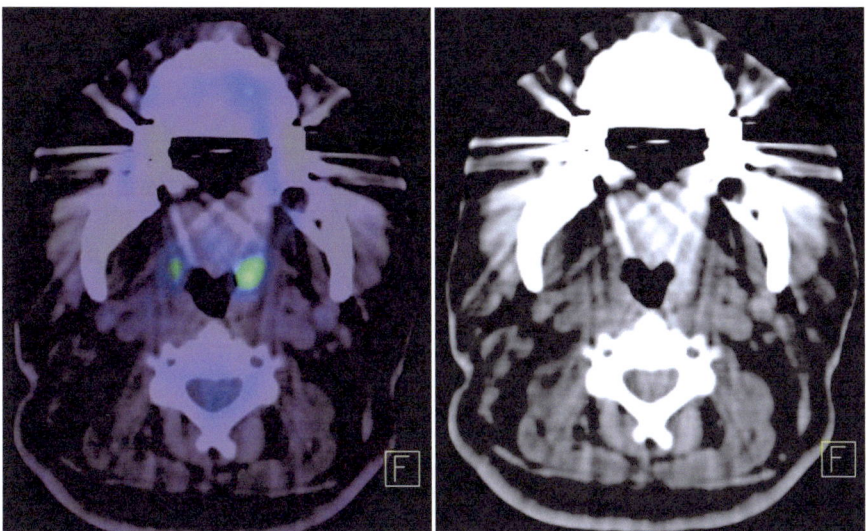

Fig. 6.1 Beam hardening artefacts due to dental fixtures

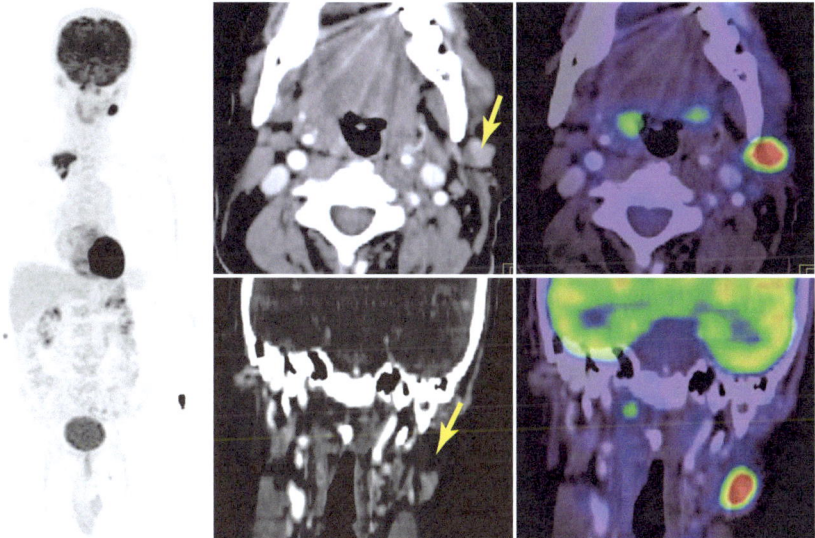

Fig. 6.2 Incidentally detected intensely FDG concentrating well-defined enhancing lesion in the left parotid gland (yellow arrow) likely benign tumour (Warthins/pleomorphic adenoma)

Incidental pathologies have been found in 25% of PET studies performed for a range of indications [9] (Fig. 6.2). The clinical impact of incidental findings needs to be considered in the context of patient care. Reviewing previous imaging, patient's history, clinical and biochemical investigations and, often, histopathologic examination may all be required to enable confident analysis of a lesion. An awareness of the incidence of these pathologies in the local population is essential. Decisions on

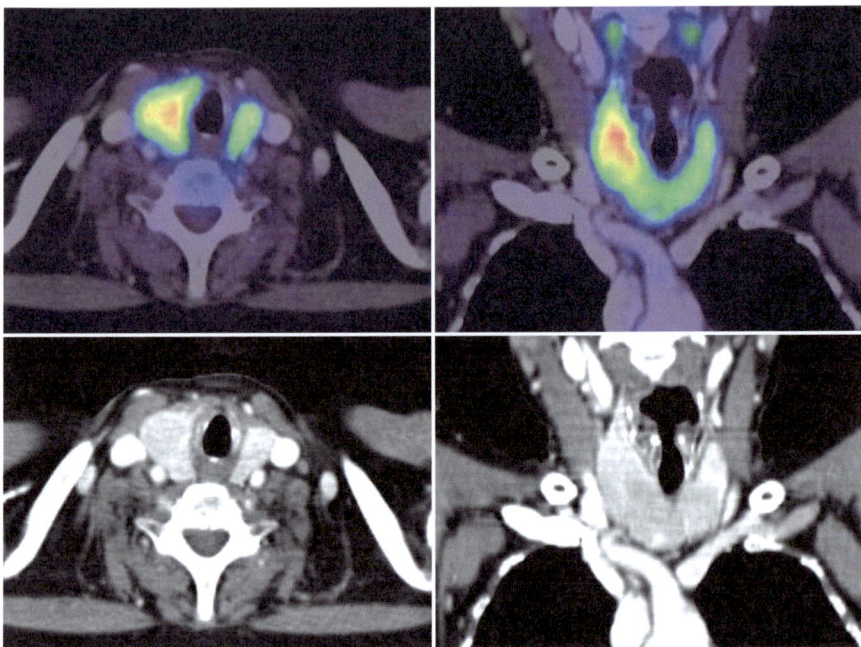

Fig. 6.3 Diffusely increased heterogeneous FDG uptake in asymmetrically enlarged (R > L) lobes of the thyroid gland

the most appropriate patient management are often enlightened by a multidisciplinary review.

In the context of known thyroid malignancy, focal thyroid uptake at the primary lesion relates to lesion size and pathological subtype [10]. Incidental uptake at other sites within the thyroid should also be treated with suspicion and, if clinically relevant, should be further assessed at US and with fine-needle aspiration cytology [11].

Increased uptake throughout the thyroid (Fig. 6.3) may represent a benign thyroiditis and may correlate with subclinical autoimmune thyroiditis and relevant auto-antibodies or may be associated with Graves' disease [12]. Thyroiditis may also involve one or more areas of the thyroid gland sparing the rest of the gland and hence warrants caution while interpreting relatively focal FDG uptake involving the part of the thyroid gland (Fig. 6.4).

Following surgery to the thyroid gland, residual uptake in the thyroid bed and related to the surgical approach, uptake in the lateral/central compartments of neck can persist for 6–12 months [13]. Routinely FDG PET/CT imaging is delayed for at least 3 months following surgery, though low-level uptake is often seen, usually quite uniformly distributed throughout the surgical bed. Foreign material, e.g. surgical stitch, can cause a granulomatous reaction and result in very localised intense activity, which can be precisely correlated to the surgical material on the CT. False-positive uptake can also be caused by recent intervention, for example, nodal biopsy or procedures like tracheostomy (Fig. 6.5). Clear clinical information and multidisciplinary discussion can help to clarify this situation.

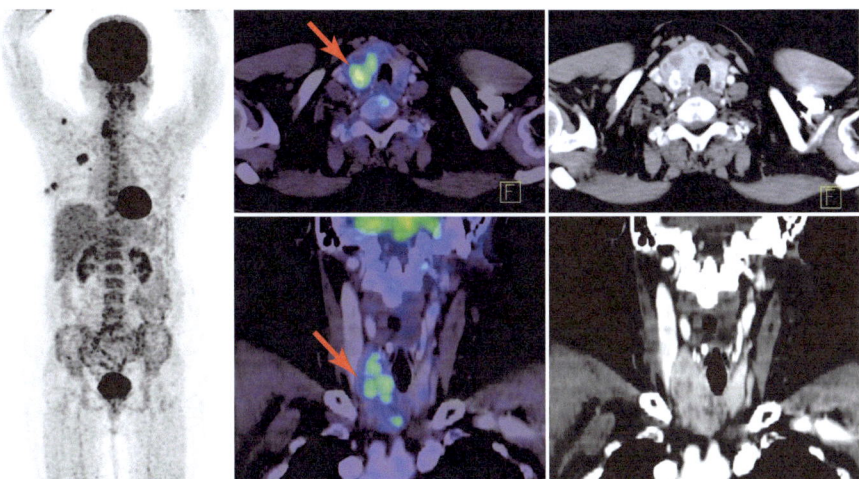

Fig. 6.4 A case of bilateral breast carcinoma. FDG PET/CT revealed moderate heterogeneous FDG-avid hypodense lesions in the enlarged right lobe of the thyroid gland. She underwent bilateral mastectomy with right hemithyroidectomy, and frozen section was done which revealed thyroiditis in the right lobe. Hence surgery was restricted to right hemithyroidectomy, and final histopathology confirmed it to be thyroiditis

6.2.3 Head and Neck: Variants, Artefacts and Pitfalls

Normal variant head and neck uptake is routinely seen on Table 6.2. FDG uptake at the salivary glands can be moderate but is generally quite symmetrical [14] (Fig. 6.6). Localised intense uptake within the parotid gland is usually interpreted as benign, related to pleomorphic adenoma or Warthin's tumour [15], though the parotid gland can contain lymph nodes (Fig. 6.7) and in the assessment of the thyroid malignancy should be dismissed with caution (Fig. 6.8). Rarely parotid metastasis has also been reported (Fig. 6.9). Review of previous or follow-up imaging is often helpful; alternatively, if there is ongoing uncertainty, definitive assessment is with ultrasound-directed biopsy or fine-needle aspiration cytology. Increased FDG accumulation can also be seen in granulomatous disorders of the salivary glands, such as sarcoidosis, where they tend to be bilateral, symmetrical and often related to typical features in the chest [16].

Muscular uptake in the head and neck region is a common finding due to muscle activation. Uptake at the floor of mouth, localising to genioglossus muscle, is a common finding and relates to normal muscle tone from maintaining upper airway patency in the supine position [17]. Physiological FDG uptake is often seen in the floor of the mouth and can be identified from the symmetry and absence of morphological changes in CT (Fig. 6.10). Uniform arytenoid and vocal cord activity is related to phonation during the uptake period (Fig. 6.11) and can be limited by maintaining a quiet, restful uptake area. Rarely pathological uptake can be present in the vocal cord region and can be identified by the asymmetry and presence of morphologically identifiable lesion in CT (Fig. 6.12). Uptake in the musculature of

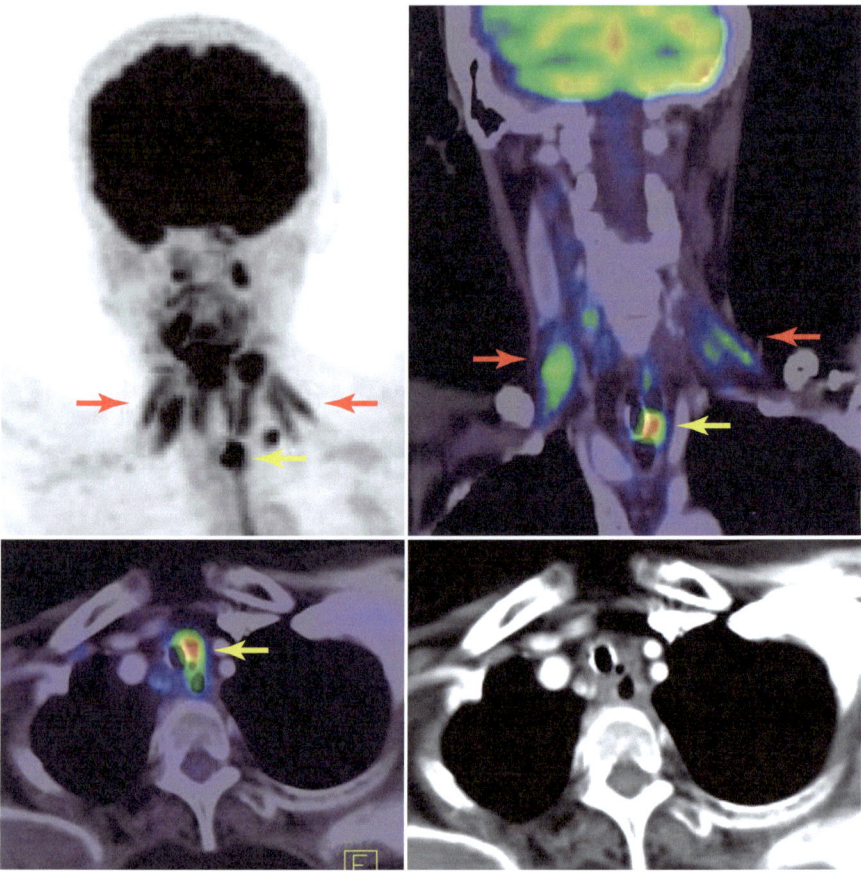

Fig. 6.5 A case of oropharyngeal carcinoma posttreatment with tracheostomy tube in situ. Note the near symmetrical intense FDG uptake in bilateral strap muscles of the neck (red arrows). Surrounding the tracheostomy tube, reactive FDG uptake is noted (yellow arrow) with no morphological abnormalities in CT part

the neck is a not infrequent finding, commonly at the longus coli/longus capitis muscles at the anterior cervical spine (Figs. 6.5, 6.13, and 6.14). This can be minimised by ensuring patient comfort during the uptake and imaging periods. Altered local muscle dynamic as a result of previous neck dissection or nerve palsy can cause marked asymmetry in the degree of muscular and also vocal cord uptake; usually close correlation with the CT study and clinical history can allow the reporter to dismiss this as a benign pitfall.

Lymphoid activation at Waldeyer's ring is a frequent finding and can be intense; it is normally symmetrical, though asymmetry can be seen as a normal variant [18] (Fig. 6.15). Particularly in the context of morphological abnormality, asymmetric activity can mimic incidental squamous tumour or lymphoma. Dedicated local imaging can help to evaluate further, though direct inspection may be required.

Table 6.2 Common variant and incidental pathology in the assessment of the head and neck region with ^{18}F-FDG PET/CT

	Appearance	Cause	Comment
Waldeyer's ring	Variable, may be intense, usually symmetrical	Physiological but may be increased secondary to URTI	Common variant
Salivary gland	Low grade can be increased in systemic inflammatory disorders	Physiological	Usually symmetrical
Parotid	Focal single or multiple FDG avid lesions. Frequently correspond with soft tissue density lesions identifiable on CT	Most commonly benign pleomorphic adenoma or Warthin's tumour	The parotid also contains lymphatic tissue. US-guided biopsy should be considered
Brown fat	Involves neck and occasionally paraspinal and retroperitoneal fat	Thermogenesis may be particularly prominent in winter	Ensure a suitably warm uptake area
Thyroid focal	FDG-avid lesion within the thyroid, which may relate to hypo-, iso- or hyperdense CT lesion	Represents an incidental thyroid malignancy in approximately 1/3 of cases [11]	Focal lesion should be assessed with US and FNAC
Thyroid diffuse	Diffusely increased thyroid uptake	May be normal variant or represent thyroiditis	Correlation with thyroid biochemistry
Vocal cord	Variable. Usually moderate and symmetric	Due to phonation during uptake period	Caution with unilateral vocal cord palsy

Uptake within thermogenic (brown) fat is usually limited to the cervical regions but can extend to paraspinal and even retroperitoneal regions [19] (Fig. 6.16). The symmetry and CT appearances are typical, and generally this is straightforward to recognise. This can be minimised by maintaining patient warmth prior to and during the PET acquisition [20].

The more common sites of thyroid metastases to the lung and bone [21] are well evaluated with ^{18}F-FDG PET/CT. FDG uptake at new or morphologically evolving pulmonary nodules usually represents metastatic disease, though this can be mimicked by a variety of benign pathologies as a result of local immunologic response. In the UK, bacterial pneumonia, tuberculosis, inflammatory conditions, radiation pneumonitis, pneumoconiosis, cryptogenic organising pneumonia, pleurodesis and eosinophilic granuloma are more often seen, though in some communities cryptococcosis, paragonimiasis or histoplasmosis are increasing in prevalence [22]. Often the characteristic morphology will suggest a benign cause. Further medical and radiological review can also help to identify these inflammatory causes. FDG-avid emboli from paravenous injections of FDG are relatively rare and usually can be recognised due to the lack of CT correlate [23].

Confidence in the diagnosis of skeletal metastases can be improved with close review of the morphology of the FDG-avid focus. Thyroid metastases to the bone are typically multiple, lytic and well defined, occasionally with an extra-osseous soft tissue component and increase in size with time.

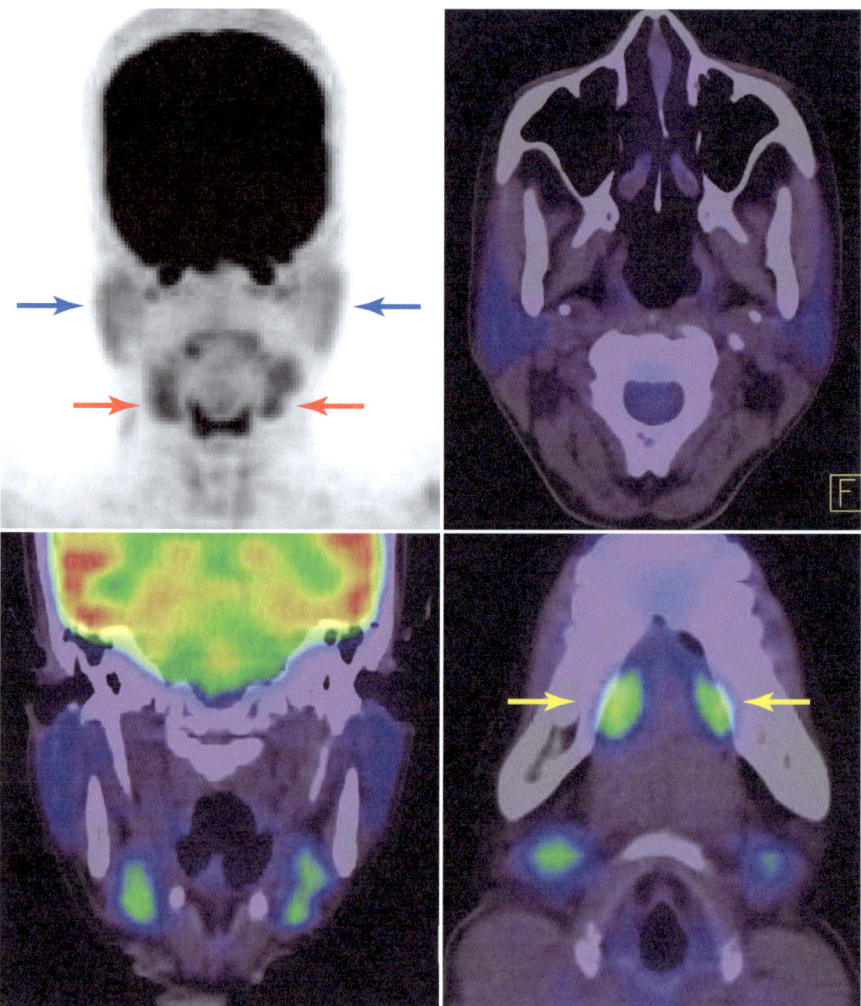

Fig. 6.6 Physiological tracer uptake in bilateral submandibular (red arrows) and parotid (blue arrows) glands. Also note the physiological tracer uptake in the mylohyoid muscles (yellow arrows)

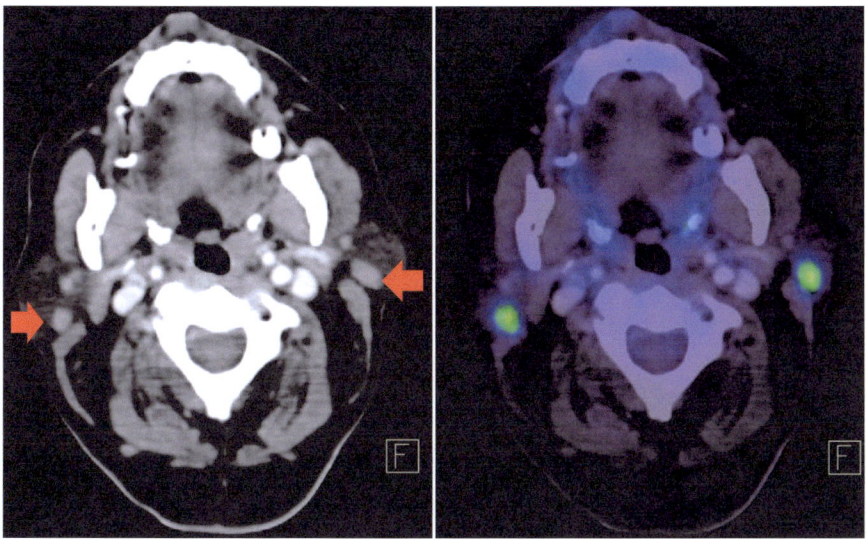

Fig. 6.7 Moderate focal FDG uptake in bilateral intra-parotid lymph nodes

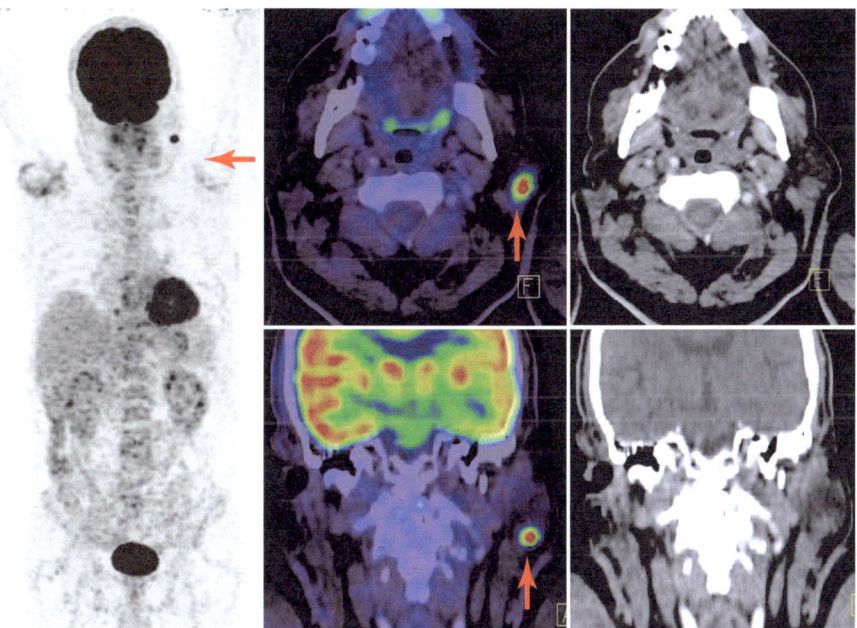

Fig. 6.8 FDG PET/CT done for evaluation of disease status in a TENIS (thyroglobulin-elevated negative iodine scan) patient showing focal intense FDG uptake in a homogeneously enhancing well-defined lesion in the left parotid gland (red arrow)

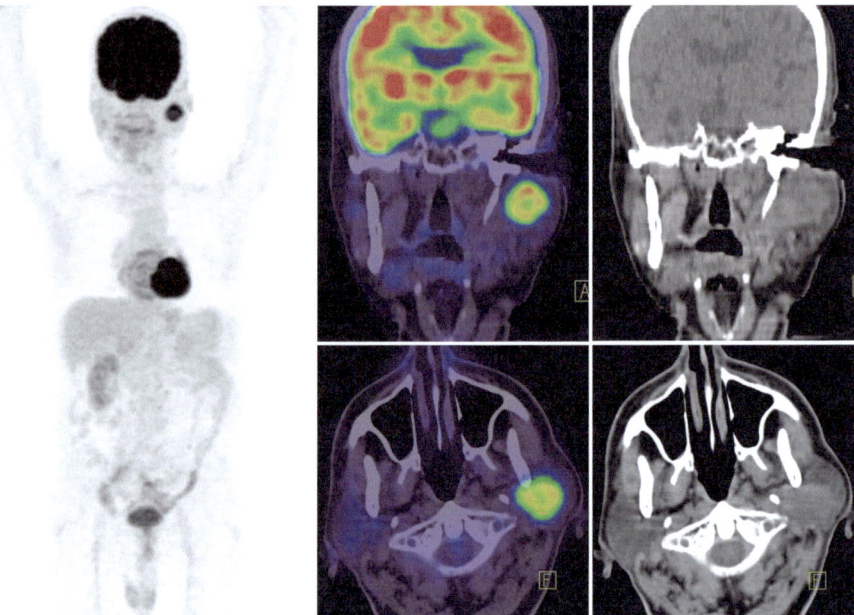

Fig. 6.9 FDG PET/CT scan done for suspected recurrence evaluation in a treated case of left renal cell carcinoma. Intensely FDG-concentrating large lesion in the left parotid which was later confirmed as metastasis

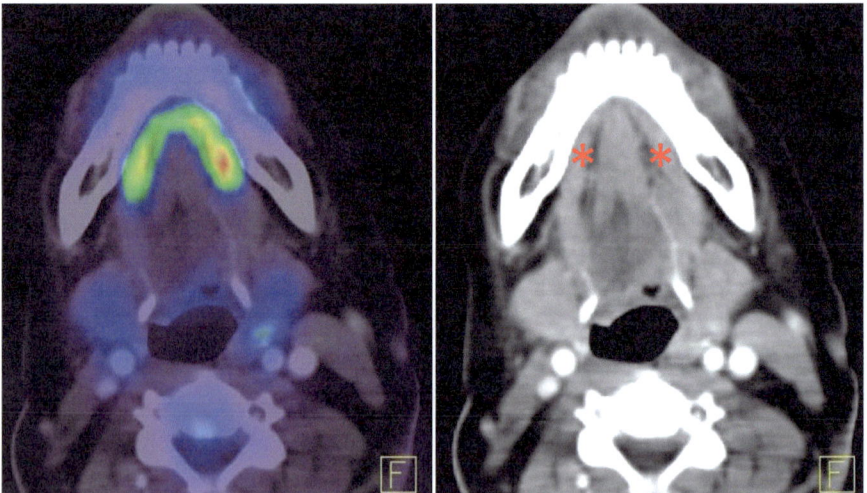

Fig. 6.10 Symmetrical physiologic uptake in the floor of the mouth (mylohyoid muscle) marked as asterisk

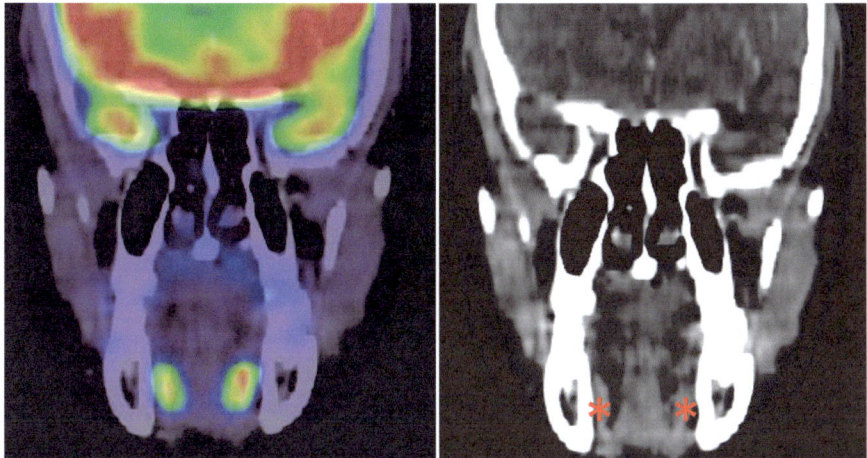

Fig. 6.10 (continued)

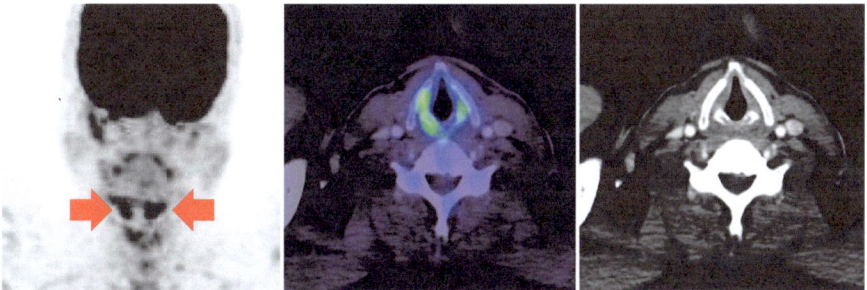

Fig. 6.11 Symmetrical FDG uptake in bilateral vocal cords (no morphological changes in CT part)

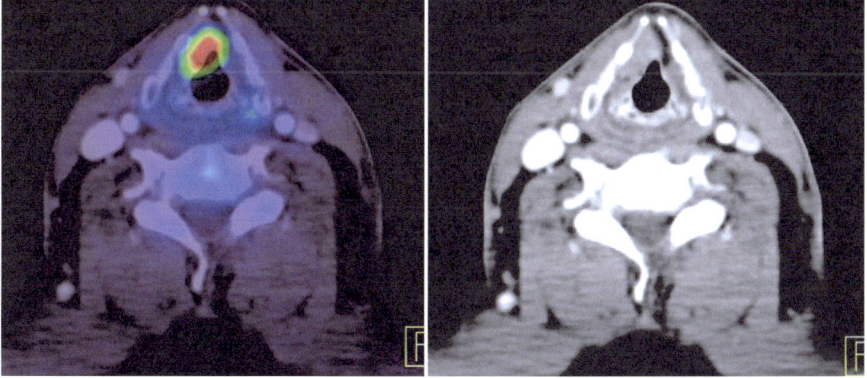

Fig. 6.12 Focal abnormal intense FDG uptake is noted in an ill-defined nodular thickening at the right false vocal cord. Note the nature of difference in pathological and physiological tracer uptake in the region of vocal cords and the associated CT changes

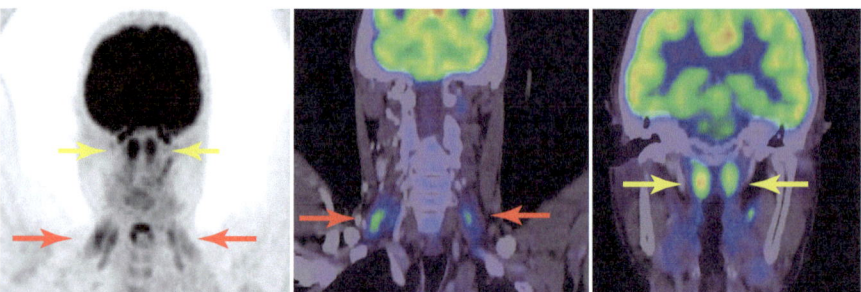

Fig. 6.13 Symmetrical FDG uptake in the strap muscles of the neck (red arrows) and in longus capitis muscle (yellow arrows)

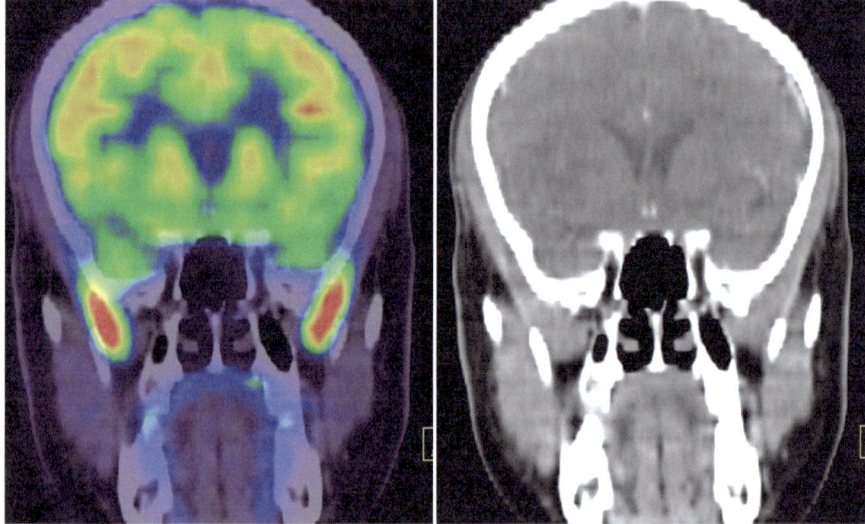

Fig. 6.14 Symmetrical intense FDG uptake in bilateral pterygoid muscles due to muscle activity

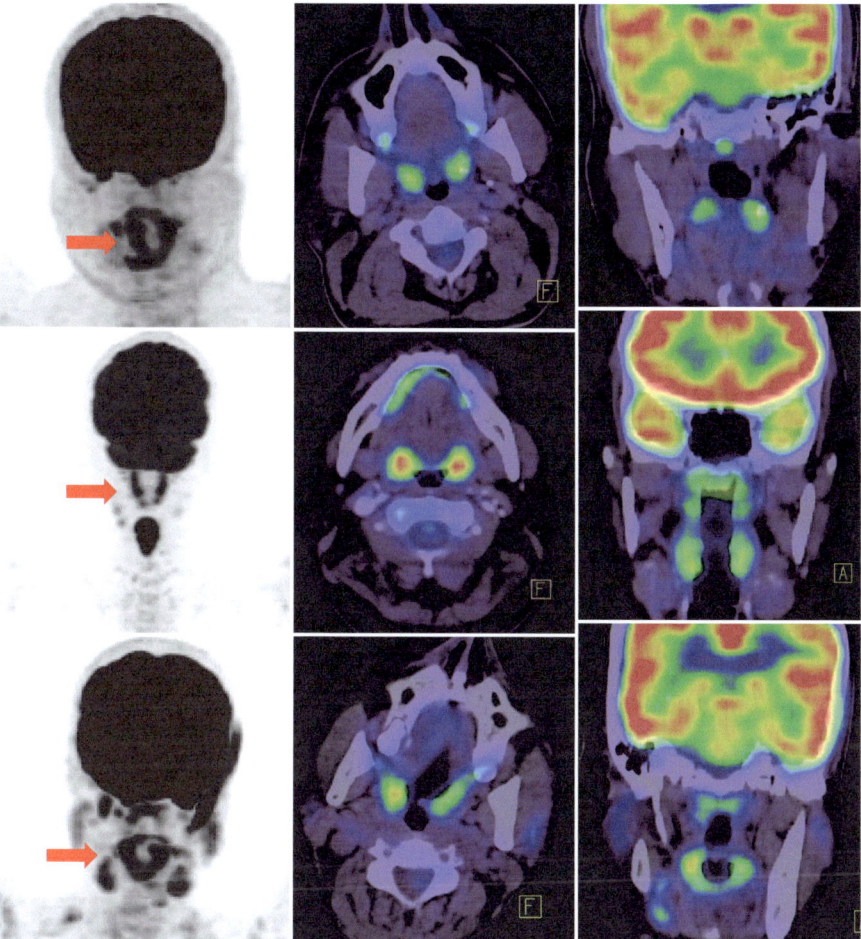

Fig. 6.15 Different patterns of FDG uptake in the Waldeyer's ring of lymphoid tissues (bold red arrows) in three different patients

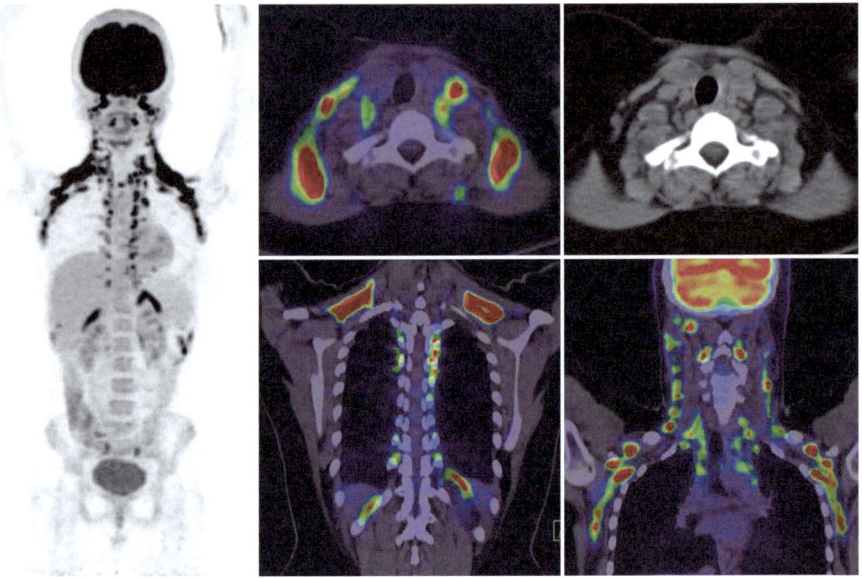

Fig. 6.16 Extensive brown fat uptake in a 19-year-old case of papillary carcinoma thyroid (TENIS). Brown fat uptake is noted in bilateral cervical, shoulders, paravertebral and retrocrural regions

Key Points

- In the context of known thyroid malignancy, focal thyroid uptake at the primary lesion relates to lesion size and pathological subtype.
- Diffuse increased uptake throughout the thyroid may represent a benign thyroiditis and may correlate with subclinical autoimmune thyroiditis and relevant auto-antibodies or may be associated with Graves' disease.
- Following surgery to the thyroid, residual uptake in the thyroid bed and related to the surgical approach can persist for 6–12 months.
- Routine FDG PET/CT imaging is delayed for at least 3 months following surgery.
- The common sites of thyroid metastases to the lung and bone are evaluated with ^{18}F-FDG PET/CT.
- FDG uptake at new or morphologically evolving pulmonary nodules usually represents metastatic disease.
- Thyroid metastases to the bone are typically multiple, lytic and well defined, occasionally with an extra-osseous soft tissue component and increase in size with time.

References

1. Barrington S, Scarsbrook A: Evidence based indications for the use of PET-CT in the UK. Royal College of Physicians, 2013
2. Corrigan AJ, Schleyer PJ, Cook GJ. Pitfalls and artifacts in the use of PET/CT in oncology imaging. Semin Nucl Med. 2015;45:481–99.
3. Culverwell AD, Scarsbrook AF, Chowdhury FU. False-positive uptake on 2-[18F]-fluoro-2-deoxy-D-glucose(FDG) positron-emission tomography/computed tomography (PET/CT) in oncological imaging. Clin Radiol. 2011;66:366–82.
4. Purohit BS, Ailianou A, Dulguerov N, Becker CD, Ratib O, Becker M. FDG-PET/CT pitfalls in oncological head and neck imaging. Insights Imaging. 2014;5(5):585–602.
5. Cook GJR, Fogelman I, Maisey MN. Normal physiological and benign pathological variants of 18-FDG PET scanning: potential for error in interpretation. Semin Nucl Med. 1996;26:308–14.
6. Delbeke D, Coleman RE, Guiberteau MJ, et al. Procedure guideline for tumour imaging with 18F-FDG PET/CT 1.0. J Nucl Med. 2006;47(5):885–95.
7. Boellaard R, O'Doherty MJ, Weber WA, et al. FDG PET and PET/CT: EANM procedure guidelines for tumour PET imaging: version 1.0. Eur J Nucl Med Mol Imaging. 2010;37(1):181–200.
8. Shreve PD, Anzai Y, Wahl RL. Pitfalls in oncologic diagnosis with FDG PET imaging: physiologic and benign variants. Radiographics. 1999;19:61–77.
9. Metser U, Miller E, Lerman H, et al. Benign non-physiologic lesions with increased 18F-FDG uptake on PET/CT: characterization and incidence. Am J Roentgenol. 2007;189:1203–10.
10. Are C, Hsu JF, Ghossein RA, Schoder H, Shah JP, Shaha AR. Histological aggressiveness of fluorodeoxyglucose positron-emission timigram (FDG-PET)-detected incidental thyroid carcinomas. Ann Surg Oncol. 2007;14(11):3210–5.
11. Soelberg KK, Bonnema SJ, Brix TH, Hegedüs L. Risk of malignancy in thyroid incidentalomas detected by (18)F-fluorodeoxyglucose positron emission tomography: a systematic review. Thyroid. 2012;22(9):918–25.
12. Yasuda S, Shohtsu A, Ide M, et al. Chronic thyroiditis: diffuse uptake of FDG at PET. Radiology. 1998;207(3):775–8.
13. Liu Y. Orthopaedic surgery-related benign uptake on FDG-PET: case examples and pitfalls. Ann Nucl Med. 2009;23:701–8.
14. Nakamoto Y, Tatsumi M, Hammoud D, et al. Normal FDG distribution patterns in the head and neck: PET/CT evaluation. Radiology. 2005;234:879–85.
15. Lee SK, Rho BH, Won KS. Parotid incidentaloma identified by combined 18F-fluorodeoxyglucose whole-body positron emission tomography and computed tomography: findings at gray-scale and power Doppler ultrasonography and ultrasound-guided fine-needle aspiration biopsy or core biopsy. Eur Radiol. 2009;19:2268–74.
16. Criado E, Sánchez M, Ramírez J, Arguis P, de Caralt TM, Perea RJ, Xaubet A. Pulmonary sarcoidosis: typical and atypical manifestations at high-resolution CT with pathologic correlation. Radiographics. 2010;6:1567–86.
17. Abouzied M, Crawford E, Nabi H. 18F-FDG imaging: pitfalls and artifacts. J Nucl Med Technol. 2005;33:145–55.
18. Heusner TA, Hahn S, Hamami ME, et al. Incidental head and neck (18)F-FDG uptake on PET/CT without corresponding morphological lesion: early predictor of cancer development? Eur J Nucl Med Mol Imaging. 2009;36:1397–406.
19. Hany TF, Gharehpapagh E, Kamel EM, Buck A, Himms-Hagen J, von Schulthess GK. Brown adipose tissue: a factor to consider in symmetrical tracer uptake in the neck and upper chest region. Eur J Nucl Med Mol Imaging. 2002;29(10):1393–8.
20. Barrington SF, Maisey MN. Skeletal muscle uptake of Fluorine-18-FDG: Effect of oral diazepam. J Nucl Med. 1996;37:1127–9.
21. Disibio G, French SW. Metastatic patterns of cancer: results from a large autopsy study. Arch Pathol Lab Med. 2008;132(6):931–9.
22. Chang JM, Lee HJ, Goo JM, et al. False positive and false negative FDG-PET scans in various thoracic diseases. Korean J Radiol. 2006;7(1):57–69.
23. Hany TF, Heuberger J, Schulthess GK. Iatrogenic FDG foci in the lungs: A pitfall of PET image interpretation. Eur Radiol. 2003;13:2122–7.

Metabolic PET/CT Imaging in Thyroid Cancer

7

Ioan Prata

Contents

7.1	Introduction	61
7.2	Primary Diagnosis/Staging	62
	7.2.1 [^{18}F]-FDG-PET/CT Scanning	62
	7.2.2 ^{124}I PET/CT Scanning	63
	7.2.3 Other Tracers Used in PET/CT Scanning	63
7.3	Response Assessment	64
References		66

7.1 Introduction

The positron emission tomography (PET) and its hybrid version PET/CT imaging, which combines morphological information obtained by the CT component with functional data provided by PET, play an important role in the evaluation and management of thyroid cancer. For many years, the primary clinical application of [^{18}F]-fluorodeoxyglucose-PET (FDG-PET) scanning in thyroid cancer was to localize disease in Tg-positive (>10 ng/mL), RAI scan-negative patients [1]. However, nowadays, the indications of the technique is steadily increasing, due to the new positron-emitting tracers available on the market, like iodine-124, ^{18}F-dihydroxyphenylalanine (^{18}F-DOPA), and gallium-68-somatostatin (68Ga-SMS) analogs, and also because of a better understanding of the physiopathological mechanisms of the thyroid cancer.

The most used tracer today is the [^{18}F]-FDG, a glucose analog labeled with the positron-emitting radioactive isotope fluorine-18. The tracer gives information

I. Prata
Bradford Teaching Hospitals NHS Foundation Trust, Bradford, United Kingdom
e-mail: prataioan@yahoo.com

© Springer International Publishing AG, part of Springer Nature 2018
S. Vinjamuri (ed.), *PET/CT in Thyroid Cancer*, Clinicians' Guides to Radionuclide Hybrid Imaging, https://doi.org/10.1007/978-3-319-71846-0_7

about cellular metabolism, which is very useful especially in poorly differentiated and more aggressive thyroid tumors.

Iodine-124, a proton-rich isotope produced in a clinical cyclotron facility, follows the same pathway as the rest of the iodine isotopes, providing information about the iodine metabolism.

[^{18}F]-DOPA, which explores amino acid uptake, decarboxylation, and storage and [68Ga]-SMS, which gives information about somatostatin receptor expression, are used in the medullary thyroid cancer [2].

7.2 Primary Diagnosis/Staging

7.2.1 [^{18}F]-FDG-PET/CT Scanning

Using FDG-PET imaging, Feine et al. [3] observed that differentiated thyroid tumors with iodine avidity have low glucose metabolism in most patients. Reciprocally, high glucose metabolism signifies a poorer tumor differentiation and higher possible malignant potential. That is the main reason why low-risk patients with differentiated thyroid cancer (DTC) are very unlikely to require a PET scanning as part of initial staging [4].

Current additional clinical uses of ^{18}F-FDG-PET scanning may include:

- Initial staging of high-risk patients with poorly differentiated thyroid cancers unlikely to concentrate RAI in order to identify sites of disease that may be missed with RAI scanning and conventional imaging
- Initial staging of invasive or metastatic Hürthle cell carcinoma
- As a powerful prognostic tool for identifying which patients with known distant metastases are at highest risk for disease-specific mortality
- Adverse histology (e.g., columnar cell, tall cell, and insular variants)

FDG-PET scans are most useful in high-risk patients, in which tumors are more biologically aggressive, and for metastatic disease. Apart from aiding in diagnosis, PET measurement of glucose metabolism provides biologic information, as noted in the standardized uptake value (SUV). Patients whose cancers take up FDG well are not likely to respond to radioactive iodine. Furthermore, the FDG-PET SUV is a strong predictor of adverse prognosis, with higher SUVs indicating worse overall prognosis [1]

There is a big interest in defining the role of [^{18}F]-FDG-PET and PET/CT in histologically non-diagnostic or inconclusive thyroid nodules in fine needle aspiration biopsy. A recent meta-analysis revealed that [^{18}F]-FDG-PET or PET/CT showed a high sensitivity in detecting cancer in patients with indeterminate FNAB results. Further examinations, such as hemithyroidectomy, were strongly recommended when a FDG-avid lesion was detected [5].

Sometimes [^{18}F]-FDG-PET or PET/CT reveals thyroid incidental uptake (TIU) of the tracer which may have a focal or a diffuse pattern. Diffuse TIU at [^{18}F]-FDG-PET or PET/CT can be considered at low risk of malignancy, being more likely associated with thyroiditis or diffuse thyroid autonomy. Approximately one-third of the focal uptakes are malignant [6]; therefore there is a recommendation that all thyroid incidentalomas will need further investigation and clinical evaluation. A dual-point PET/CT was not observed to be beneficial in discriminating benign from malignant lesions.

7.2.2 ^{124}I PET/CT Scanning

Several iodine isotopes such as ^{123}I, ^{125}I, and ^{131}I play an important role in nuclear medicine, both for diagnostic purposes and for therapy. Iodine-^{124} is a positron-emitting isotope of iodine and therefore suitable PET imaging, which has a half-life of 4.2 days.

The main initial interest in ^{124}I PET exams is its role in estimating the functional volume of the thyroid as opposed to the anatomical volume of the gland. In this respect, ^{124}I PET has been proven to be superior to both high-resolution ultrasound and planar scintigraphy using other isotopes of iodine [7].

Iodine-124 has recently been used for staging of differentiated thyroid cancer, but for now there are mainly small series of patients or case reports, but the results are good, with ^{124}I-PET being considered a promising technique to improve treatment planning in thyroid cancer. It is particularly valuable in patients suffering from advanced differentiated thyroid cancer prior to radioiodine therapy and in patients with suspected recurrence and potential metastatic disease [8]. In combination with the high resolution PET technique and the possibilities to combine with CT it could lead to improved clinical decision-making [9].

A further potential application of ^{124}I PET is in the management of patients with differentiated thyroid cancer. ^{131}I whole-body scans lack anatomical resolution and are recognized as being false negative in some patients with metastatic disease. ^{124}I PET has theoretical advantages over ^{131}I in such patients [10].

7.2.3   Other Tracers Used in PET/CT Scanning

[^{18}F]-DOPA has been used in an attempt to increase the PET scan sensibility in primary detection and staging of medullary thyroid carcinoma. Although the studies were on limited number of patients, some of the authors claimed that ^{18}F-DOPA PET is a useful supplement to morphological diagnostic imaging, improving lymph node staging and enabling a more specific diagnosis of primary tumor [11]. With all the promising initial evidence, the [^{18}F]-DOPA PET or PET/CT was not included in the guidelines for management of differentiated thyroid cancer for the initial tumor and staging assessment.

In recent studies, **[68Ga]-SMS** has been used as a tracer in thyroid cancer. It has been demonstrated that well-differentiated thyroid cancer (WDTC) cells have a high expression of Sstr2, Sstr3, and Sstr5. The results show that using somatostatin tracers will not lead to any significant difference in tumor detection [12]; however this should be taken into consideration in view of assessing Sst analogs for peptide receptor radionuclide therapy [13].

7.3 Response Assessment

The most valuable role of **^{18}F-FDG-PET** and PET/CT in the work-up of differentiated thyroid cancer is in those patients who present with increasing serum thyroglobulin (Tg) levels and a negative diagnostic radioiodine whole-body scan post-thyroidectomy, according to the American Thyroid Association (ATA) guidelines.

Approximately one-third of patients with differentiated thyroid cancers will have tumor recurrences. Distant metastases are present in about 20% of patients with recurrent cancer. The loss of the ability to concentrate radioiodine and produce thyroglobulin is a sign of dedifferentiation, which occurs in about 30% of patients with persistent or recurrent thyroid cancer. Dedifferentiation is associated with poorer responses to conventional therapy and difficulty monitoring tumor burden [14].

A recent study highlights that thyroid cancer dedifferentiation is characterized by glucose transporter (GLUT1) upregulation and reduced expression of sodium iodide symporter (NIS) [15]. This is the main reason why the [^{18}F]-FDG is such an important tool in the follow-up of thyroid cancer.

Also it is worth mentioning the limitation of the anatomical imaging techniques (ultrasonography and CT/MR scans) in patients already operated and treated with iodine.

The usefulness of [^{18}F]-FDG-PET may depend on factors, such as Tg level, TSH stimulation by thyroid hormone withdrawal, and TSH stimulation by rhTSH administration. It is accepted nowadays that FDG-PET is more useful at Tg levels over 10 ng/mL [16].

The American Thyroid Association recommended in the Guidelines for Patients with Thyroid Nodules and Differentiated Thyroid Cancer the use of [^{18}F]-FDG-PET in the following situations:

- As a powerful prognostic tool for identifying which patients with known distant metastases are at highest risk for disease-specific mortality
- As a selection tool to identify those patients unlikely to respond to additional RAI therapy
- As a measurement of posttreatment response following external beam irradiation, surgical resection, embolization, or systemic therapy

Recently, **[^{124}I]-PET** has emerged as a valuable diagnostic tool for the detection of recurrent or residual DTC disease, and the data afforded are helpful in the planning of therapy during follow-up of DTC patients.

[^{124}I]-PET imaging may offer a higher sensitivity than the conventional [^{131}I] scan because the spatial resolution is greater. Moreover, the use of combined PET/CT (computed tomography) scanners allows thyroid cancers to be imaged using a high-resolution PET technique. This may increase the clinical application of such imaging in thyroid cancer patients because detailed anatomical information is obtained and iodine-positive tissue can be located [17]. Unfortunately, although promising, there is yet little experience and not enough studies up-to-date, causing some authors to conclude this is just a more expensive way to image with radioiodine and no clear clinical advantage has been shown [18].

In patients with medullary thyroid cancer, ^{18}F-FDG-PET positivity seems to be associated with biochemical progressive disease (calcitonin and CEA-increasing serum levels) and significantly affects survival. **[18]F-DOPA** PET seems to be more important in assessing the extent of the disease in patients with residual disease, whereas ^{18}F-FDG-PET can more accurately identify patients with progressive disease [19]. Both scans are useful complementary imaging tools for accurate identification of metastases both in MTC patients with occult disease and in MTC patients with more aggressive disease. Accurate detection of metastatic disease is a prerequisite for tailoring further treatment, which might be further surgery, pretargeted radioimmunotherapy, or multikinase inhibitor treatment [20].

Key Points

- Differentiated thyroid tumors with iodine avidity have low glucose metabolism in most patients.
- High glucose metabolism signifies a poorer tumor differentiation and higher possible malignant potential.
- FDG-PET scans are most useful in high-risk patients, in which tumors are more biologically aggressive, and for metastatic disease.
- Diffuse increased FDG-PET in the thyroid is more likely associated with thyroiditis or diffuse thyroid autonomy.
- Approximately one-third of the focal increased tracer uptake within the thyroid are malignant.
- All thyroid incidentalomas will need further investigation and clinical evaluation.
- The most valuable role of ^{18}F-FDG-PET is in the work-up of differentiated thyroid cancer in patients with increasing serum thyroglobulin (Tg) levels and a negative diagnostic radioiodine scan.
- The loss of the ability to concentrate radioiodine and produce thyroglobulin is a sign of dedifferentiation.
- The usefulness of [^{18}F]-FDG-PET often depends on Tg level, TSH stimulation by thyroid hormone withdrawal, and TSH stimulation by rhTSH administration.
- In patients with medullary thyroid cancer, ^{18}F-FDG-PET positivity seems to be associated with biochemical progressive disease (calcitonin and CEA-increasing serum levels) and significantly affects survival.

References

1. Larson SM, Robbins R. Positron emission tomography in thyroid cancer management. Semin Roentgenol. 2002;37:169–74.
2. Treglia G, Giovanella L, Rufini V. PET and PET/CT imaging in thyroid and adrenal diseases: an update. Hormones (Athens). 2013;12(3):327–33.
3. Feine U, Lietzenmayer R, Hanke JP, et al. Fluorine-18-FDG and iodine-131-iodide uptake in thyroid cancer. J Nucl Med. 1996;37(9):1468–72.
4. American Thyroid Association (ATA) Guidelines Taskforce on Thyroid Nodules and Differentiated Thyroid Cancer, Cooper DS, Doherty GM, Haugen BR, et al. Revised American Thyroid Association management guidelines for patients with thyroid nodules and differentiated thyroid cancer. Thyroid. 2009;19:1189.
5. Wang N, Zhai H, Yingli L. Is fluorine-18 fluorodeoxyglucose positron emission tomography useful for the thyroid nodules with indeterminate fine needle aspiration biopsy? A meta-analysis of the literature. J Otolaryngol Head Neck Surg. 2013;42:38.
6. Bertagna F, Treglia G, Piccardo A, Giubbini R. Diagnostic and clinical significance of F-18-FDG-PET/CT thyroid incidentalomas. J Clin Endocrinol Metab. 2012;97:3866–75.
7. Frey P, Townsend D, Jeavons A, Donath A. In vivo imaging of the human thyroid with a positron camera using I-124. Eur J Nucl Med. 1985;10(9-10):472–6.
8. Freudenberg LS, Antoch G, Jentzen W, Pink R, Knust J, Gorges R, et al. Value of 124I-PET/CT in staging of patients with differentiated thyroid cancer. Eur Radiol. 2004;14:2092–8.
9. Phan HT, et al. The diagnostic value of 124I-PET in patients with differentiated thyroid cancer. Eur J Nucl Med Mol Imaging. 2008;35:958–65.
10. McDougall IR, Davidson J, Segall GM. Positron emission tomography of the thyroid, with an emphasis on thyroid cancer. Nucl Med Commun. 2001;22:485–92.
11. Hoegerle S, Altehoefer C, Ghanem N, Brink I, Moser E, Nitzsche E. 18F-DOPA positron emission tomography for tumour detection in patients with medullary thyroid carcinoma and elevated calcitonin levels. Eur J Nucl Med. 2001;28(1):64–71.
12. Ambrosini V, Rubello D, Nanni C, Al-Nahhas A, Fanti S. 68Ga-DOTA-peptides versus 18F-DOPA PET for the assessment of NET patients. Nucl Med Commun. 2008;29(5):415–7.
13. Ocak M, Demirci E, Kabasakal L, Aygun A, Tutar RO, Araman A, Kanmaz B. Evaluation and comparison of Ga-68 DOTA-TATE and Ga-68 DOTA-NOC PET/CT imaging in well-differentiated thyroid cancer. Nucl Med Commun. 2013;34(11):1084–9.
14. Sturgeon C, Angelos P. Identification and treatment of aggressive thyroid cancers. Oncology (Williston Park). 2006;20(3):253–60.
15. Grabellus F, Nagarajah J, Bockisch A, Schmid KW, Sheu SY. Glucose transporter 1 expression, tumor proliferation, and iodine/glucose uptake in thyroid cancer with emphasis on poorly differentiated thyroid carcinoma. Clin Nucl Med. 2012;37(2):121–7.
16. Ruiz Franco-Baux JV, Borrego Dorado I, Gómez Camarero P, Rodríguez Rodríguez JR, Vázquez Albertino RJ, Navarro González E, Astorga JR. F-18-fluordeoxyglucose positron emission tomography on patients with differentiated thyroid cancer who present elevated human serum thyroglobulin levels and negative I-131 whole body scan. Rev Esp Med Nucl. 2005;24(1):5–13.
17. Lee J, Nah KY, Kim RM, Oh YJ, An YS, Yoon JK, An GI, Choi TH, Cheon GJ, Soh EY, Chung WY. Effectiveness of [124I]-PET/CT and [18F]-FDG-PET/CT for localizing recurrence in patients with differentiated thyroid carcinoma. J Korean Med Sci. 2012;27(9):1019–26.
18. Buscombe JR. Radionuclides in the management of thyroid cancer. Cancer Imaging. 2007;7:202–9.
19. Verbeek HH, et al. Clinical relevance of 18F-FDG PET and 18F-DOPA PET in recurrent medullary thyroid carcinoma. J Nucl Med. 2012;53(12):1863–71.
20. Kauhanen S, et al. Complementary roles of 18F-DOPA PET/CT and 18F-FDG PET/CT in medullary thyroid cancer. J Nucl Med. 2011;52(12):1855–63.

Benign and Malignant Thyroid Diseases on ^{18}F FDG PET/CT: Pictorial Atlas

8

Haseeb Ahmed and Hosahalli Mohan

Contents

8.1	Case 1	68
	8.1.1 Normal Thyroid	68
8.2	Case 2	69
	8.2.1 Focal Increased FDG Uptake in the Thyroid Gland	69
8.3	Case 3	70
	8.3.1 Nodular Goiter	70
8.4	Case 4	71
	8.4.1 Nodular Goiter	71
8.5	Case 5	72
	8.5.1 Multinodular Goiter	72
8.6	Case 6	73
	8.6.1 Multinodular Goiter with Hurthle Cell Change	73
8.7	Case 7	74
	8.7.1 Incidental Papillary Thyroid Cancer	74
8.8	Case 8	75
	8.8.1 Incidental Medullary Thyroid Cancer	75
8.9	Case 9	76
	8.9.1 Papillary Thyroid Cancer with Reactive Lymph Node in the Neck	76
8.10	Case 10	77
	8.10.1 I^{131} Positive and ^{18}F FDG PET/CT Negative	77
8.11	Case 11	78
	8.11.1 I^{131} Negative and ^{18}F FDG PET/CT Positive	78

H. Ahmed (✉) · H. Mohan
Guy's and St. Thomas' NHS Foundation, Great Maze Pond, London, SE1 9RT UK
e-mail: haseeb1400@gmail.com

© Springer International Publishing AG, part of Springer Nature 2018
S. Vinjamuri (ed.), *PET/CT in Thyroid Cancer*, Clinicians' Guides to Radionuclide Hybrid Imaging, https://doi.org/10.1007/978-3-319-71846-0_8

8.12 Case 12... 79
   8.12.1 Progression on Tyrosine Kinase Inhibitor.................. 79
8.13 Case 13... 80
   8.13.1 Stable on Tyrosine Kinase Inhibitor 80
8.14 Case 14... 81
   8.14.1 Incidental Lung Carcinoma............................. 81
8.15 Case 15... 82
   8.15.1 Thyroid Carcinoma with Incidental Thymoma.............. 82

The FDG-PET/CT has no a clear role in the preoperative evaluation for differentiated thyroid cancer patients.

Diffuse FDG uptake in the thyroid gland is associated with benign conditions such as thyroiditis, nodular goiter, and Graves' disease.

The prevalence of focal uptake varied between 0.1 and 4.8% in various studies.

The prevalence of thyroid cancer in these lesions was 36% and varied from 10 to 64% in different reports.

8.1 Case 1

8.1.1 Normal Thyroid

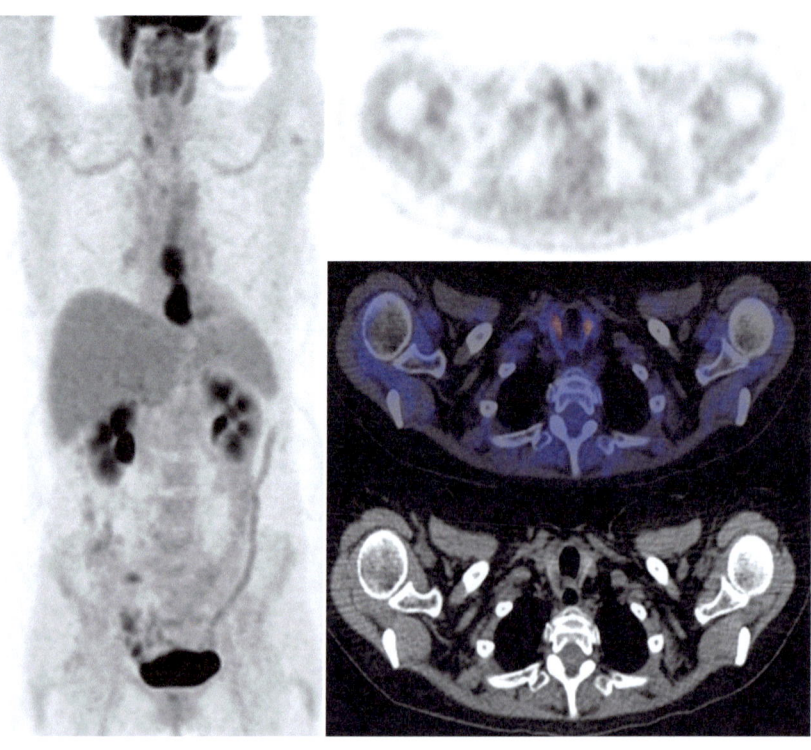

Clinical details: A 54-year-old female with primary esophageal cancer.

There is increased tracer uptake within the esophagus in keeping with known esophageal cancer. There is symmetrical, low-grade homogeneous tracer uptake within the thyroid.

Teaching Point
Physiological thyroid uptake is usually symmetrical, homogeneous, and low grade.

8.2 Case 2

8.2.1 Focal Increased FDG Uptake in the Thyroid Gland

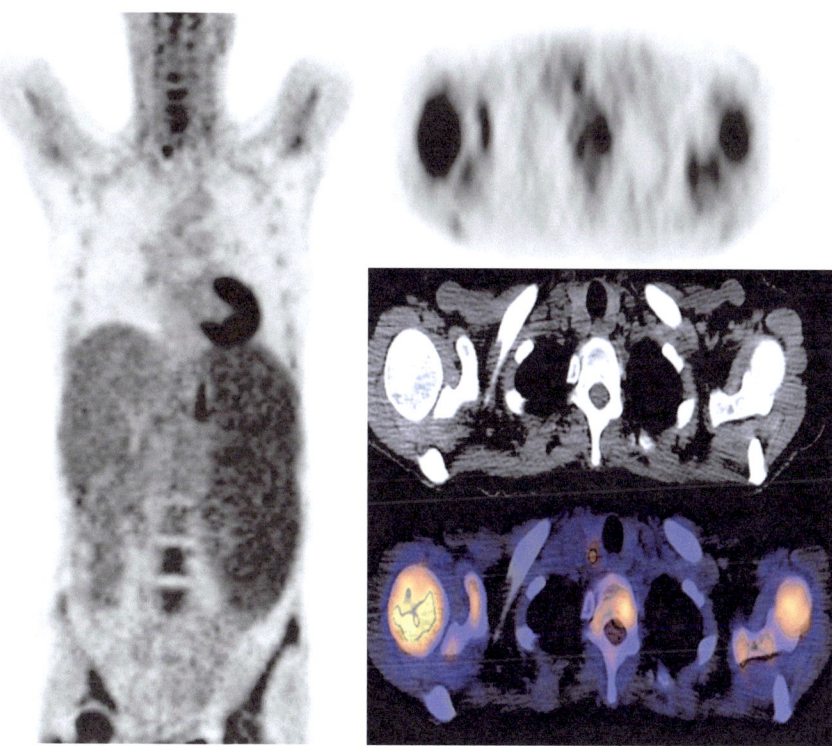

Clinical history: A 48-year-old patient who underwent a PET/CT for workup of polycythemia now progressed to myelofibrosis.

There is focal low-grade FDG uptake in the right lobe of the thyroid which was subjected to FNA and diagnosed to be a benign colloid nodule Thy 2.

Teaching Points
Focal or diffuse FDG uptake in the thyroid is often seen as an incidental finding.

Reported incidence of thyroid incidentalomas with increased FDG uptake is 1.2–2.3% on PET examinations.

Focal uptake in the thyroid gland can be benign or malignant. Any focal thyroid uptake warrants further workup with FNA to confirm or exclude sinister pathology.

8.3 Case 3

8.3.1 Nodular Goiter

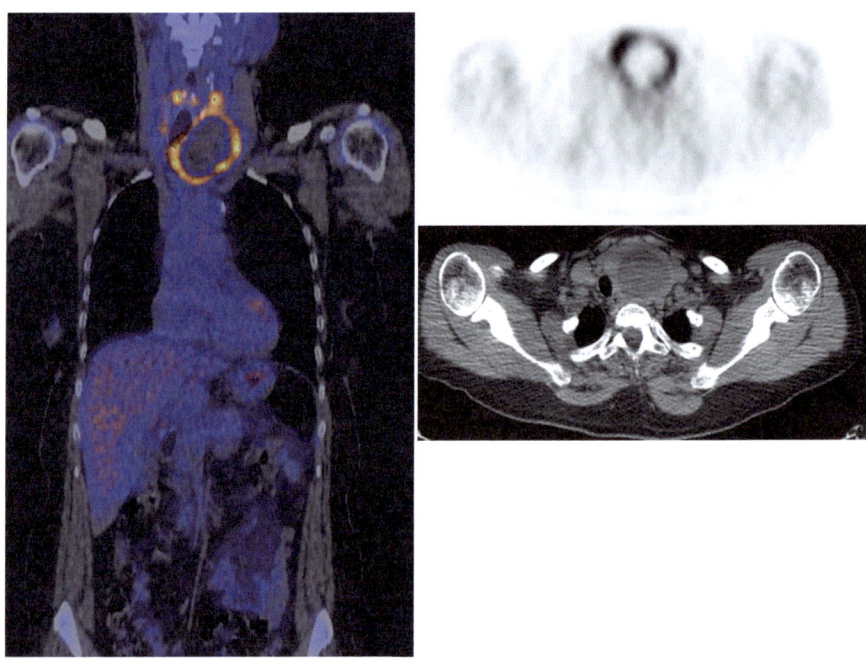

Clinical history: A 59-year-old female with a history of carcinoma of the lung with incidental thyroid uptake. There is a large neck mass with a rim of FDG uptake around the periphery with reduced uptake in the center of the mass. On FNA, the lesion was diagnosed as colloid cyst Thy 2c.

Teaching Points
Variant of benign thyroid uptake.
A rim of activity with cold center can be a presentation of a colloid cyst or a large simple cyst.

8.4 Case 4

8.4.1 Nodular Goiter

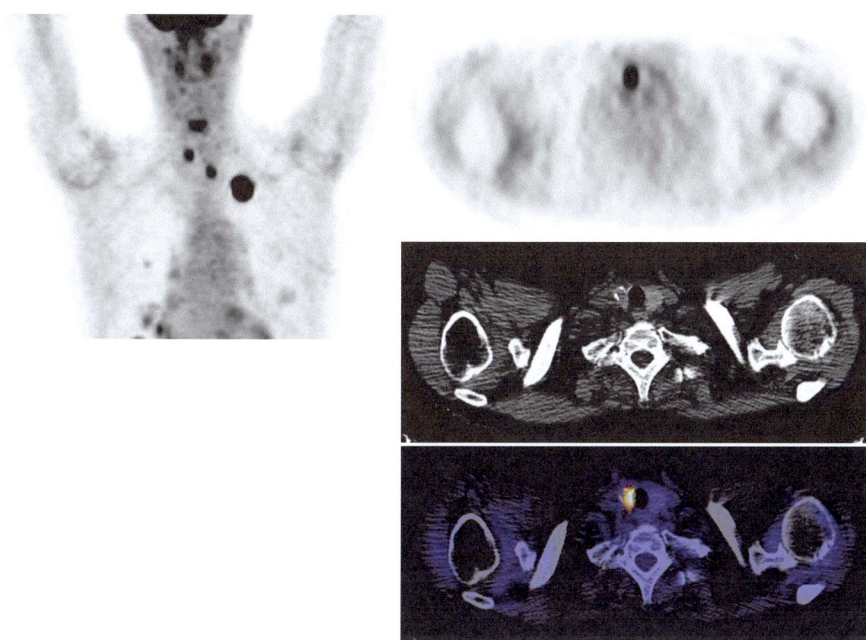

Clinical details: A 66-year-old female with a history of lung carcinoma. The staging PET/CT showed abnormal increased tracer uptake within the lung mass and mediastinal lymph nodes. There is an incidental focal thyroid uptake with focal calcification within the right lobe of the thyroid. FNA of the right thyroid nodule showed Thy 2.

Teaching Point
Benign thyroid nodules can also demonstrate significantly increased tracer uptake.

8.5 Case 5

8.5.1 Multinodular Goiter

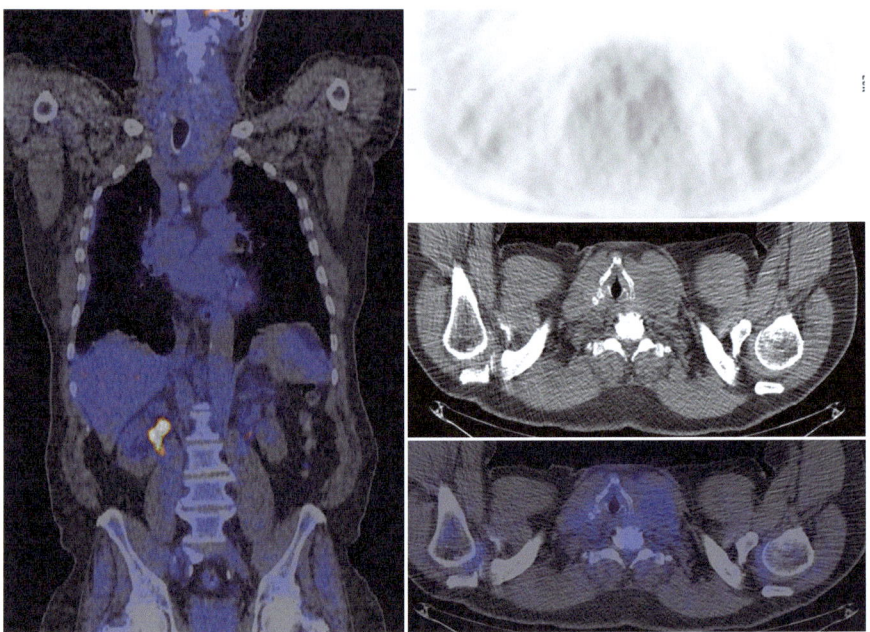

Clinical details: An 88-year-old male who underwent a staging PET/CT for carcinoma of the lung. The scan shows a bulky multinodular goiter with no focal or diffuse increased tracer uptake. FNA was not performed as the scan appearance is typical of a multinodular goiter.

Teaching Points
Multinodular goiter shows heterogeneous tracer uptake and can be large enough to cause compression of the trachea, esophagus, and adjacent structures.

8.6 Case 6

8.6.1 Multinodular Goiter with Hurthle Cell Change

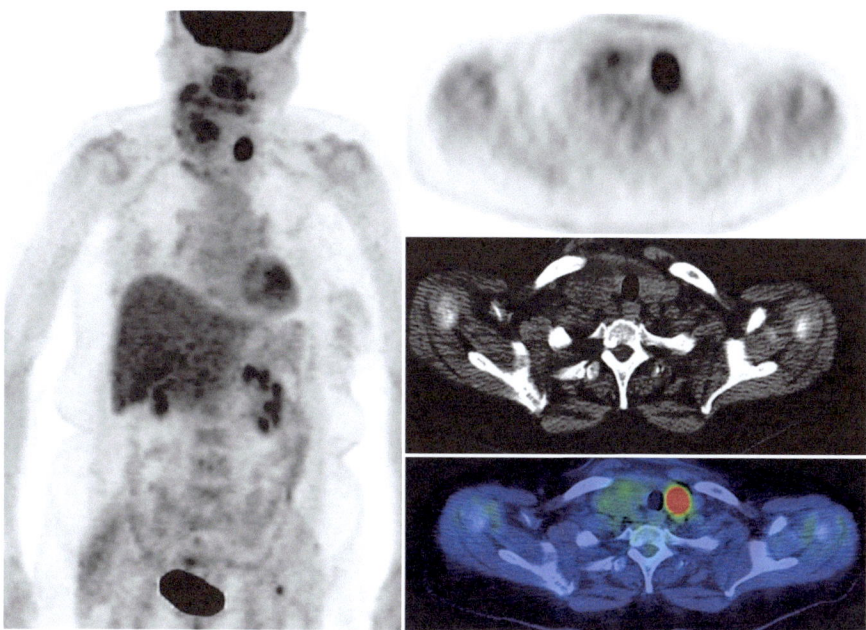

Clinical details: A 74-year-old male who underwent ^{18}F FDG PET/CT scan for a suspected squamous cell carcinoma or lymphoma. The ^{18}F-FDG PET/CT scan shows a focal avid tracer uptake within the left thyroid lobe. The FNA was suggestive of Hurthle cell neoplasm Thy 3. A total thyroidectomy was performed, and histopathology showed Hurthle cell change on a background of MNG. No capsular or vascular invasion was noted.

8.7 Case 7

8.7.1 Incidental Papillary Thyroid Cancer

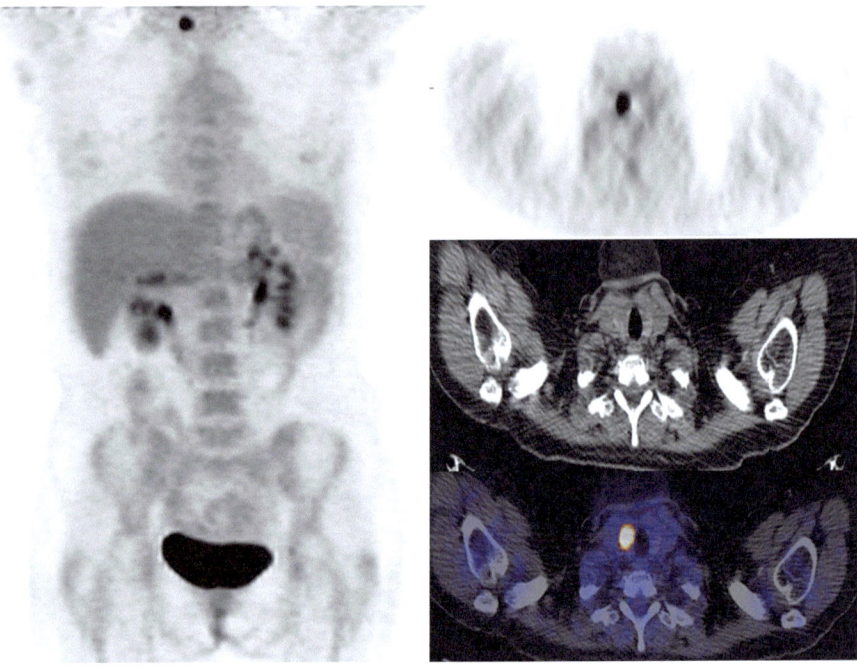

Clinical details: Patient with squamous cell carcinoma of the left tonsil presenting for restaging PET/CT after radical chemoradiation. The PET/CT scan shows increased tracer uptake within the right lobe of the thyroid, and FNA revealed papillary thyroid cancer, Thy 5. Total thyroidectomy and histopathology showed papillary thyroid carcinoma pT1a N0, encapsulated follicular variant.

Teaching Points
Increased focal thyroid uptake should be investigated with ultrasound and FNA.

8.8 Case 8

8.8.1 Incidental Medullary Thyroid Cancer

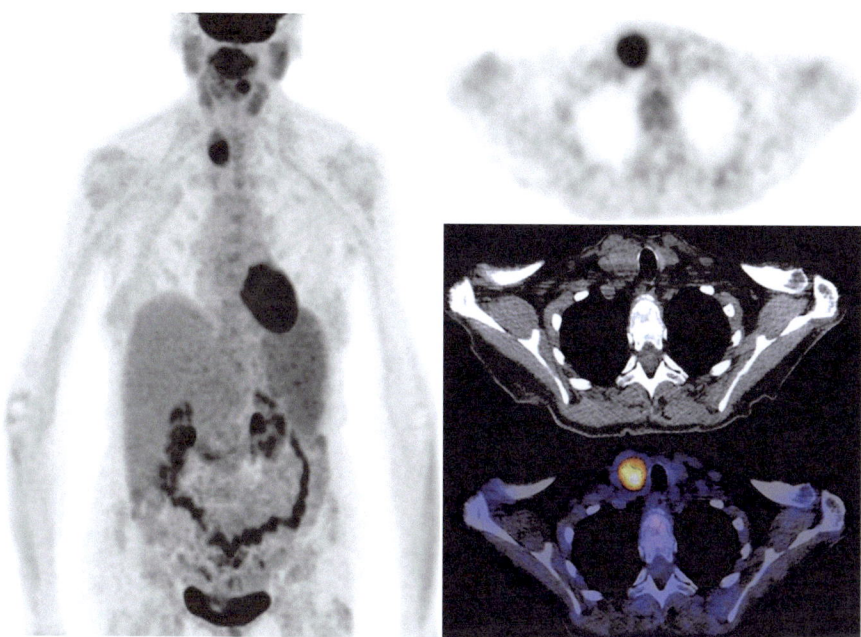

Clinical details: An 80-year-old female with relapsed splenic marginal zone lymphoma. Previous treatment with R-CVP chemotherapy in 2012. The patient relapsed in 2014 with progression in 2015. The PET/CT scan shows a focal increased tracer uptake within the right lobe of the thyroid. The FNA revealed medullary thyroid cancer Thy 5.

Teaching Points
Increased focal thyroid uptake should be investigated with ultrasound and FNA.

8.9 Case 9

8.9.1 Papillary Thyroid Cancer with Reactive Lymph Node in the Neck

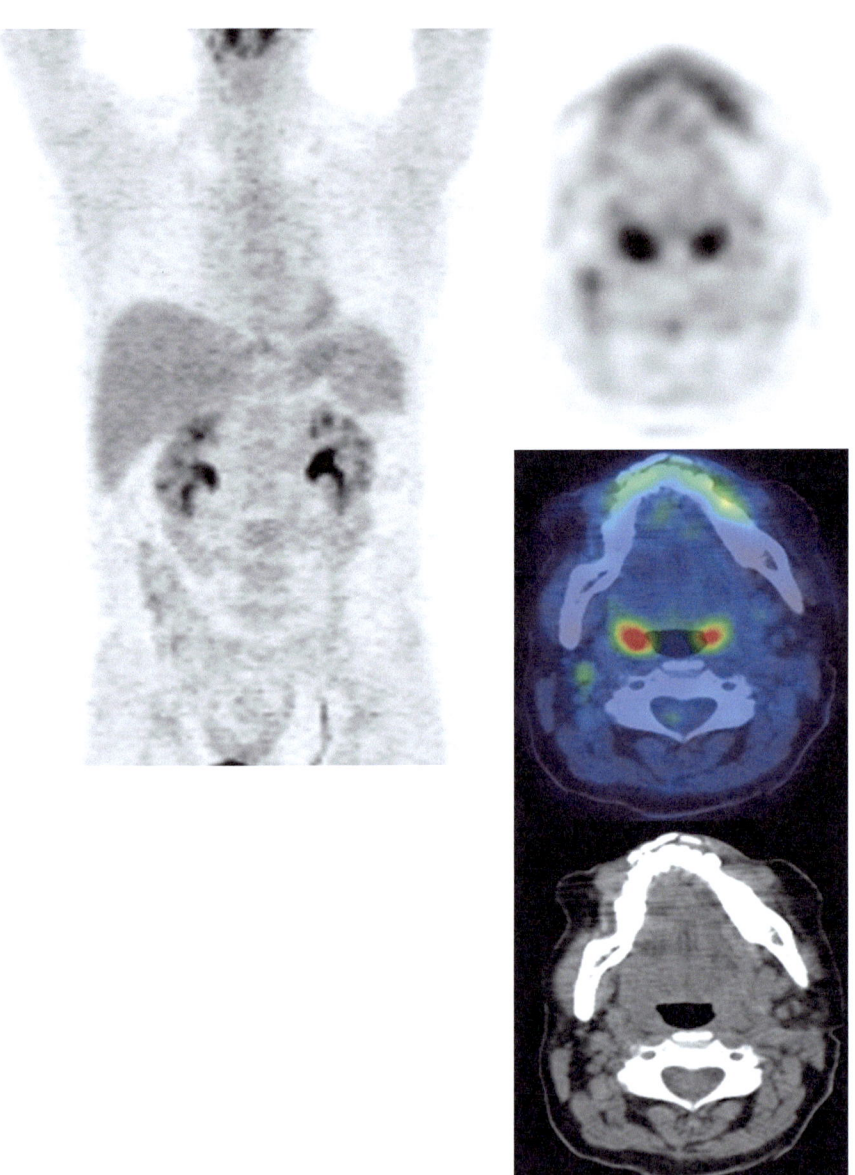

Clinical details: A 64-year-old female with papillary thyroid cancer diagnosed in 1990. The patient developed a swelling on the left side of the neck with thyroglobulin levels of 3.5. The patient underwent PET/CT which showed low-grade uptake in the right level II lymph node. The FNA of the right level II lymph node showed non-specific reactive lymph node - colloid Thy 1.

Teaching Points
In thyroid carcinoma the lymph nodes in the neck with increased FDG uptake can be due to inflammatory causes.

8.10 Case 10

8.10.1 I^{131} Positive and ^{18}F FDG PET/CT Negative

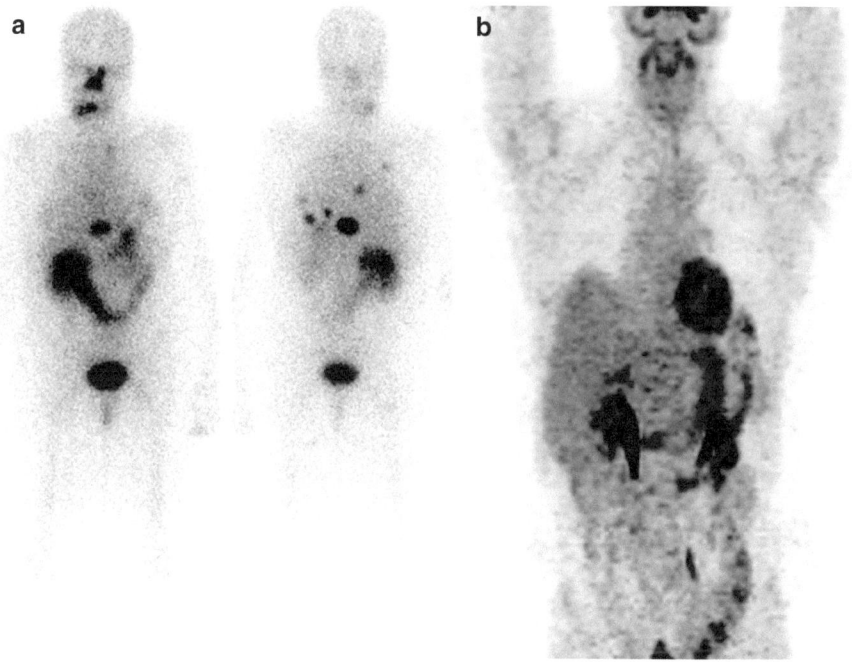

Clinical details: A 65-year-old female with follicular thyroid cancer and skeletal metastases. She underwent surgery for the T10 metastases along with radiotherapy and has had a good response with stable disease after radioiodine treatment. Her thyroglobulin level currently remains at 74 in March 2013 which is significantly reduced when compared to the previous level of 172.

Teaching Points
Differentiated thyroid carcinoma can be non-avid on ^{18}F FDG PET/CT but will show uptake on I^{131} scan.

8.11 Case 11

8.11.1 I¹³¹ Negative and ¹⁸F FDG PET/CT Positive

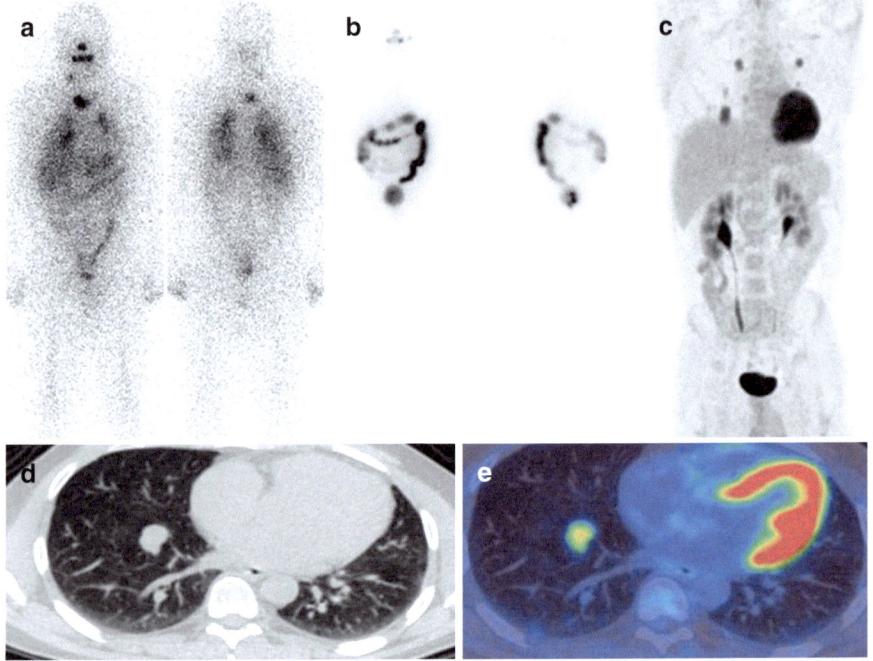

Clinical details: A 52-year-old male with follicular variant thyroid cancer diagnosed in 1999. The last radioiodine treatment was in December 2014 which did not show any iodine-avid disease within the lungs.

Teaching Points

Differentiated thyroid carcinoma can transform into undifferentiated and more aggressive form of cancer and can lose its ability to take up iodine. Such cancers will be metabolically active on ¹⁸F FDG PET/CT but will not show any uptake on I¹³¹ scan.

8.12 Case 12

8.12.1 Progression on Tyrosine Kinase Inhibitor

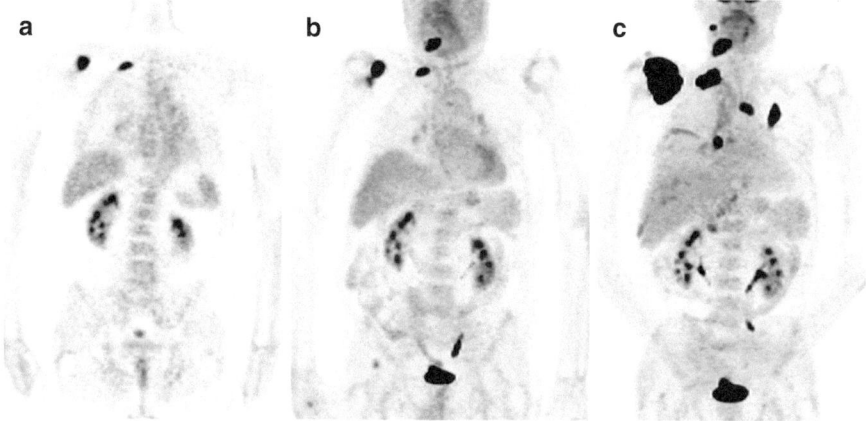

Clinical details: A 69-year-old male with recurrent papillary thyroid carcinoma with anaplastic elements. (**a**) PET/CT in August 2010 - thyroglobulin levels 0.5. There is abnormal increased tracer uptake in the right scapula, right second rib, mediastinum, and right neck lymph nodes in keeping with FDG avid progressive disease. (**b**) PET/CT in September 2011 - thyroglobulin level of 34. There is increase in FDG uptake in the pre-existing lesions in the right scapula, right second rib and mediastinum and new lesion in the neck. (**c**) PET/CT in August 2012 - thyroglobulin 451. There is further increase in the FDG uptake in the right scapula, right second rib and mediastinum with new lesions in the neck and lungs.

8.13 Case 13

8.13.1 Stable on Tyrosine Kinase Inhibitor

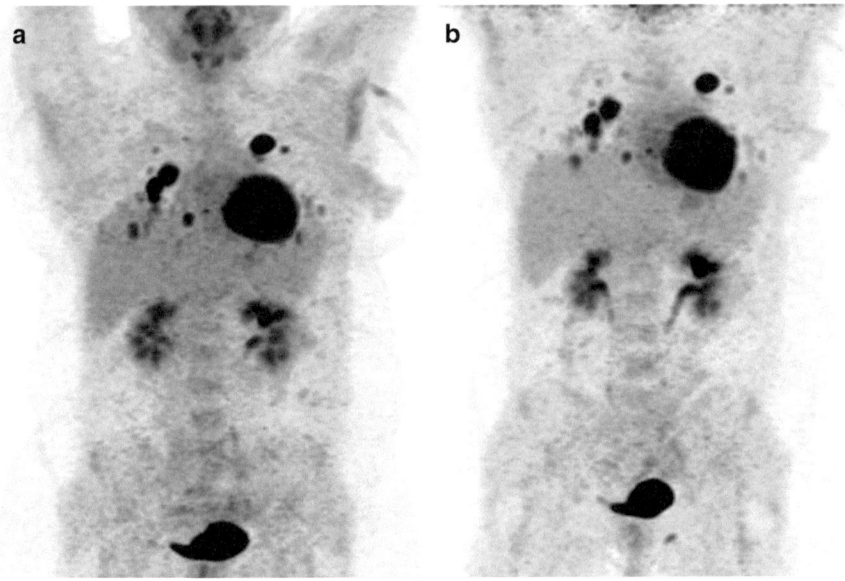

Clinical details: The patient with a diagnosis of follicular thyroid cancer, poorly differentiated, with lung metastases (**a**). She is currently on sorafenib 200 mg a day. Her lung disease remains stable on this dose (**b**).

8.14 Case 14

8.14.1 Incidental Lung Carcinoma

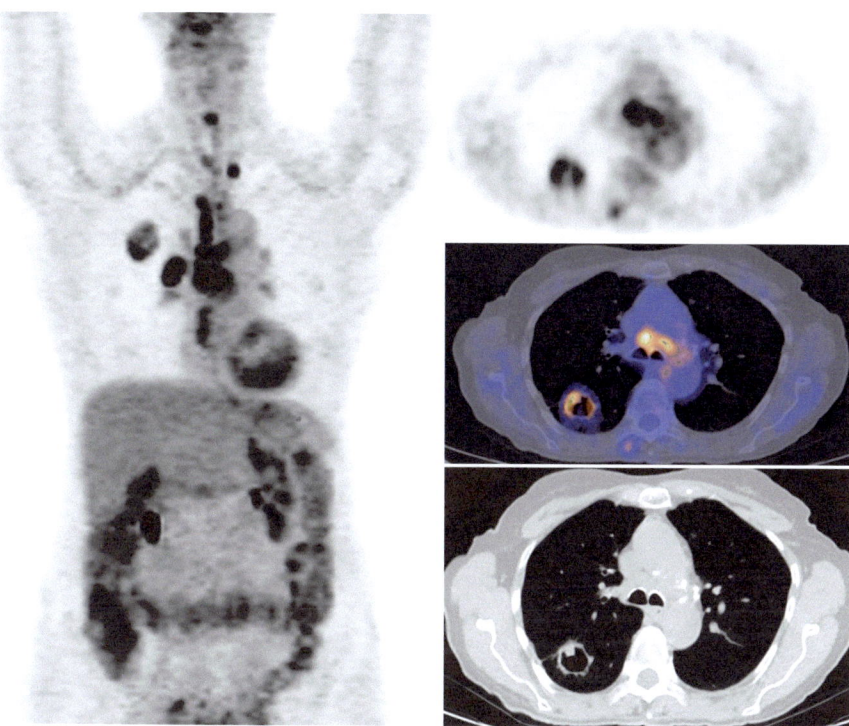

Clinical details: A 78-year-old female with papillary thyroid cancer with lung metastasis and mediastinal nodes. Incidental findings of a new lung lesion which was confirmed to be a primary lung carcinoma on biopsy.

Teaching Points
The metabolically active lung lesions on a background of a thyroid carcinoma can also be secondary to a primary lung cancer.

8.15 Case 15

8.15.1 Thyroid Carcinoma with Incidental Thymoma

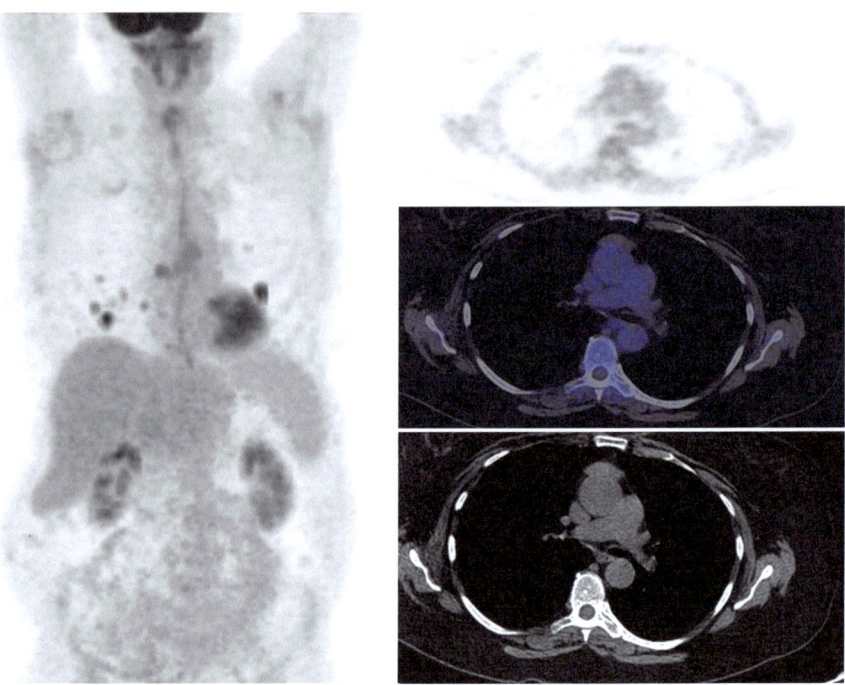

Clinical details: This is a 65-year-old lady with a previous history of papillary thyroid cancer originally diagnosed in 2001 with known lung metastases. She was treated with a total thyroidectomy and a radioactive iodine treatment. Following that she was given the all clear. She was diagnosed with myasthenia. The patient had rising thyroglobulin levels and underwent a PET/CT for restating. There was an anterior mediastinal mass which was a thymoma resulting in myasthenia.

Index

A
Ablation therapy, 39
Ablative iodine 131 therapy
 post-thyroidectomy, 29
Activated inflammatory processes, 46
American Joint Committee on Cancer (AJCC)
 classification, 28
Anaplastic carcinoma, 11, 12, 28
Anaplastic thyroid cancer, 21
Arytenoid and vocal cord activity, 49
Autoimmune thyroiditis, 21, 48

B
Benign nodules, 26
Benign thyroiditis, 48
British Association of Endocrine and
 Thyroid Surgeons (BAETS), 16
British Thyroid Association (BTA) Thyroid
 Cancer Guidelines 2014, 3, 16–19

C
Central compartment nodal disease, 18, 29
Central lymph node dissections, 16, 18
Chemotherapy, 1, 21
Clinical assessment, thyroid cancer, 2, 3, 16
Cytological diagnosis, pre-operative, 7

D
Differentiated thyroid cancer (DTC), 4, 5,
 16–20, 62, 64
Diffuse FDG uptake, 68, 69
Diffuse thyroid autonomy, 62–63
^{18}F-Dihydroxyphenylalanine (^{18}F-DOPA),
 61–63, 65
Discordant nodule, 37

Distant metastases, 17, 29
Dynamic risk stratification (DRS), 19

E
Endemic goitre, 2
Esophageal cancer, 69
Evidence-based thyroid cancer practice, 16
External beam radiotherapy (EBRT), 19–21, 41
Extrathyroidal tumour extension, 17, 26

F
Familial disease, 17
^{18}F-dihydroxyphenylalanine (^{18}F-DOPA),
 61–63, 65
^{18}F-FDG PET/CT, 64, 65
 beam hardening artefacts, 47
 bilateral breast carcinoma, 49
 bilateral intra-parotid lymph nodes, 53
 in bilateral pterygoid muscles, 56
 in bilateral vocal cords, 55
 biodistribution, 46
 brown fat uptake, 58
 FDG-avid emboli, paravenous injections, 51
 incidental pathologies, 46–48
 ^{131}I negative and ^{18}F FDG PET/CT
  positive, 78
 ^{131}I positive and ^{18}F FDG PET/CT
  negative, 77
 local CT artefacts, 46
 in longus capitis muscle, 56
 normal variant head and neck uptake, 49, 50
 patient management, 48
 patient movement, 46
 physiological tracer uptake, 52
 pulmonary nodules, 51
 renal cell carcinoma, 54

^{18}F-FDG PET/CT (cont.)
    scanning, 62–63
    strap muscles of the neck, 56
    technical problems, 46
    UK oncologic clinical practice, 45
    variant and incidental pathology, 51
    Waldeyer's ring of lymphoid tissues, 57
Fine needle aspiration cytology (FNAC) biopsy, 3, 4, 16, 26–28, 36, 62
^{18F}Fluoro-deoxy-glucose positron emission tomography (FDG PET) scan, 4
Follicular carcinoma, 10
Follicular epithelial-derived cancers, 11
Follicular-type tumours, 17
Follicular variant papillary carcinoma, 10

G
Gallium 68 peptide imaging, 29
Gallium-68-somatostatin (68Ga-SMS), 61, 63
Gamma camera planar imaging, 36
Genetic syndromes, 2
Graves' disease, 48, 68

H
Hemithyroidectomy, 10, 16, 17, 20, 21, 49, 62
High-resolution collimators, 41
Hurthle (oncocytic) cell-variant follicular tumours, 11, 17, 18, 40, 73
Hyperfunctioning thyroid nodules, 37, 39
Hypofunctioning thyroid nodule, 37, 39

I
Incidental lung carcinoma, 81
Incidental medullary thyroid cancer, 75
Incidental papillary thyroid cancer, 74
Incidental squamous tumour or lymphoma, 50
Iodine
    ^{123}I imaging, 41
    ^{124}I imaging, 61, 62
    ^{131}I MIBG imaging, 29
    ^{131}I negative and ^{18}F FDG PET/CT positive, 78
    ^{124}I PET/CT scanning, 63, 64
    ^{131}I positive and ^{18}F FDG PET/CT negative, 77
    ^{131}I radioiodine ablative therapy, 29
    ^{131}I therapy, 18, 19

K
Kim criteria, 3

L
Lateral lymph node dissections, 18
Liver function tests, 3
Lymphoid activation, Waldeyer's ring, 50

M
Malignant nodules, 26, 27
MALT lymphoma, 21
Management of Thyroid Cancer 2014 guidance, 19
Medullary and anaplastic cancers, 29, 30
Medullary thyroid cancer (MTC), 20, 21, 65
Metabolic PET/CT imaging
    anatomical imaging techniques, 64
    clinical applications, 62
    distant metastases, 64
    glucose transporter upregulation, 64
    morphological information, 61
    posttreatment response, 64
    prognostic tool, 64
    Tg level, 64
    thyroid tumors with iodine avidity, 62
    TSH stimulation, 64
Metastatic disease, 17, 18, 29, 40, 51, 62, 63, 65
Micro-medullary thyroid cancer, 20
Micro-papillary carcinomas, 17
Minimally invasive follicular carcinoma, 11, 17, 18
Mixed solid cystic lesions, 27
Modulated radiotherapy, 29
Motion artefacts, 46
Multifocal disease, 17, 28
Multinodular goiter
    heterogeneous tracer uptake, 72
    with Hurthle cell change, 73
Multiple endocrine neoplasia (MEN), 20, 29
Muscular uptake, 49
Myelofibrosis, 69

N
Neck lymph node, 2, 18, 79
Neck musculature, 49
Nodal disease and distant metastases, 26
Nodal metastases in MTC, 20, 28
Nodal staging, 28
Nodular goiter, 68, 70, 71
Non-medullary thyroid cancer, 2

O
Oncocytic tumour, , 17–18, 11
Oropharyngeal carcinoma posttreatment, 50

Index

P
Papillary cancer, 1, 9, 10, 18, 28–30
Papillary microcarcinoma, 10, 17
Papillary thyroid carcinoma, 9
    with anaplastic elements, 79
    with reactive neck node, 76
Patient-centred approach, 16
Peptide receptor radionuclide therapy, 63
Physiological thyroid uptake, 69
Poorly differentiated thyroid cancer, 11
Post-^{131}I ablation scintigraphy, 41
Post-ablation scan, 19
Pre-ablative imaging methods, 41
Pre-therapy scanning, 41
Primary tumour staging, 28
Prophylactic lateral neck lymph node dissection, 18
Prophylactic surgery, 21
Pulmonary metastases, micronodular/macronodular, 29

R
Radiation exposure, 1–2
Radio-immunotherapy, 21
Radioiodine (RAI)
    ablation, 4, 21, 41, 62, 64
    scan, 61
    therapy, 64
Radioiodine remnant ablation (RRA), 18, 19
Radio-iodine therapy, 11
Radioisotope treatment, 21
Radiological imaging
    benign nodule, 26
    incidence, 25
Radionuclide imaging
    clinical examination, 36
    evaluation and clinical management, 35
    indications, 36
Radiopharmaceuticals, 38
Radiotherapy planning, 29

S
Scintigraphy for staging/restaging, 39–41
Skeletal metastases, 51
Solitary discordant thyroid nodules, 37
Staging systems, 4, 5

T
Thyroidal tissue stunning, 41
Thyroid cytology, 4
Thyroid incidental uptake (TIU) of the tracer, 62
Thyroiditis, 48, 63, 68
Thyroid lymphoma, 21
Thyroid nodules
    goitre, 3
    hyperfunctioning, 37
    hypofunctioning, 37
Thyroid scan reporting, 37, 39
TNM staging system, 4, 5, 28
Total thyroidectomy, 17, 74
Treatment, 4, 7, 10, 16, 18–21, 28, 35, 36, 63
Tyrosine kinase inhibitor, 79, 80

U
Ultrasound, 3, 4, 16, 18, 26–30, 63
    classification system, 27
Union for International Cancer Control (UICC) classification, 28

V
Vascular follicular bone lesions, 3

W
Widely invasive follicular carcinoma, 11, 17

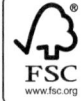

MIX
Papier aus verantwortungsvollen Quellen
Paper from responsible sources
FSC® C105338

If you have any concerns about our products,
you can contact us on
ProductSafety@springernature.com

In case Publisher is established outside the EU,
the EU authorized representative is:
Springer Nature Customer Service Center GmbH
Europaplatz 3, 69115 Heidelberg, Germany

Printed by Libri Plureos GmbH
in Hamburg, Germany